BECOME THINNER LEANER STRONGER

The basic science of muscular growth

Ronald L Abrams

Table of Contents

Take charge of your own fitness and create a regimen that will lead to exceptional fat loss and muscle building.

Chapter 21

The No-BS Guide to Supplements
Discover what's and isn't worth your money—you might be surprised.

Chapter 22

Your physique will change from here on.
You are about to embark on a journey of self transformation. Where will it take you?

Chapter 23

FAQs
Answer to to some Frequently Asked Questions about training, nutrition and lifestyle.

INTRODUCTION

Become Thinner Leaner Stronger is a fitness and nutrition book is a guide that focuses on helping individuals, particularly women, achieve their fitness goals by emphasizing a combination of weightlifting, proper nutrition, and cardiovascular exercise. The program is designed to promote fat loss, muscle development, and overall strength. It provides a structured approach to training and nutrition, making it accessible for those looking to improve their physical fitness and appearance. The book outlines workout routines, diet plans, and essential principles for achieving a lean and strong body. Bodybuilding workouts are a structured and intensive form of resistance training aimed at developing and sculpting muscle mass. These workouts focus on hypertrophy, which is the process of increasing the size of muscle fibers. Bodybuilders use a combination of weightlifting exercises, cardiovascular training, and nutrition to achieve their goals. The ultimate aim is to achieve a well-proportioned, muscular physique with low body fat. Bodybuilding workouts often involve split routines, targeting different muscle groups on different days, and progressive overload, where the resistance is gradually increased to stimulate muscle growth. These workouts require dedication, consistency, and a commitment to proper form and nutrition to achieve desired results.

WHY BECOME THINNER LEANER STRONGER IS DIFFERENT

Become Thinner Leaner Stronger stands out from other fitness programs for several reasons:

Evidence-Based Approach: The program emphasizes scientific research and evidence-based principles, which can be reassuring for individuals looking for a rational and effective approach to fitness.

Emphasis on Progressive Overload: It focuses on the concept of progressive overload, which is crucial for muscle and strength development. This means gradually increasing the weight or intensity of your workouts over time.

Balanced Approach: *Become Thinner Leaner Stronger* promotes a balanced approach to fitness, encompassing strength training, nutrition, and cardio, rather than extreme or fad-based methods.

Customizable: The program allows for customization to suit an individual's goals, whether it's building muscle, losing fat, or improving overall fitness.

Clarity and Simplicity: The book provide clear and simple guidelines, making it accessible for beginners while still being valuable for experienced gym-goers.

Emphasis on Nutrition: Nutrition is a critical component, and the book offers practical advice on how to manage your diet effectively to support your fitness goals.

Long-Term Sustainability: *Become Thinner Leaner Stronger* emphasizes creating sustainable habits and long-term fitness improvements, rather than quick fixes.

These are the things that the billionaire owners of the multi-billion dollar fitness industry would prefer you to remain ignorant of.

While it's important to be cautious about making broad claims regarding the fitness industry, there are a few things that some might argue the industry doesn't heavily promote to bodybuilders:

Sustainable Progress: The fitness industry often emphasizes quick fixes and supplements, but long-term, sustainable progress is key. Consistency, proper nutrition, and gradual increases in weight and intensity can be more effective than shortcuts.

Individual Variability: Every body is different, and what works for one person may not work for another. It's crucial for bodybuilders to understand their own unique needs and adapt their routines accordingly.

Rest and Recovery: Overtraining can be counterproductive. Sufficient rest and recovery time is vital for muscle growth and overall health, which isn't always emphasized in marketing.

Nutrition Over Supplements: While supplements can have a place in a bodybuilder's regimen, a balanced diet with real, whole foods is often more important than relying solely on supplements.

Mental Health: The mental aspect of bodybuilding is often overlooked. The industry doesn't always emphasize the importance of a healthy mindset, which is crucial for long-term success and overall well-being.

Remember that the fitness industry is diverse, and there are many reputable professionals and resources that prioritize these principles. It's essential to do your research and consult with experts who have your best interests in mind.

Chapter 1

THE UNSPOKEN OBSTACLE TO REACHING YOUR HEALTH AND FITNESS OBJECTIVES

When it comes to bodybuilding, many individuals embark on a journey with ambitious health and fitness objectives in mind. They envision sculpted physiques, increased strength, and improved overall well-being. Yet, beneath the surface of this seemingly straightforward path to success lies an unspoken obstacle that often hinders progress and leaves many aspiring bodybuilders frustrated. In this exploration, we will unveil this hidden challenge, shed light on the factors contributing to it, and provide insights on how to overcome it, ultimately helping you achieve your health and fitness goals in the world of bodybuilding.

The "Unspoken Obstacle" is a concept that highlights a common challenge people face when working towards their health and fitness objectives. It suggests that there are factors or barriers that aren't openly discussed but can significantly hinder one's progress in bodybuilding. These obstacles can include:

Unrealistic expectations: Many individuals set unattainable goals, which can lead to frustration and disappointment.

Lack of consistency: Inconsistent training and nutrition can hinder progress, as dedication and discipline are essential in bodybuilding.

Poor nutrition: A balanced diet is crucial for muscle growth and recovery, and inadequate nutrition can be a hidden obstacle.

Overtraining: Excessive exercise without adequate rest can lead to burnout, injuries, and slow progress.

Mental barriers: Self-doubt, lack of motivation, and negative self-talk can be unspoken obstacles to reaching fitness goals.

Inadequate recovery: Insufficient sleep and recovery can impair muscle growth and overall health.

Social influences: Peer pressure, societal norms, or a lack of support can affect one's ability to stay committed to their goals.

Lack of proper guidance: Not seeking advice from experienced trainers or professionals can be a hidden obstacle, as having the right knowledge is crucial in bodybuilding.

Addressing these unspoken obstacles and seeking support, guidance, and consistency are key steps in overcoming them and achieving your health and fitness objectives in bodybuilding.

Chapter 2

WHAT THE MAJORITY OF PEOPLE DON'T KNOW ABOUT HEALTH, NUTRITION AND FITNESS

PART ONE: BASIC SCIENCE OF THE BODY

The basic science of the human body is known as human physiology. It involves the study of how the body's organs and systems function, including topics like cell biology, anatomy, biochemistry, and more. Understanding the body's physiology is essential for healthcare professionals and scientists to diagnose and treat diseases, as well as for anyone interested in maintaining a healthy lifestyle.

ENERGY: 1. The capacity to do work.

2. Energy is the power recieved from electricity, fuel, food and other sources in order to work or produce motion.

3. Energy is the mental or physical strength of a person that can be directed towards some activities.

Chemistry: 1. Chemistry is the branch of science that studies the composition, structure, properties, and changes of matter. It explores how different substances interact with one another at the molecular and atomic level.

2. Chemistry is the science of matter and the transformations it undergoes. It encompasses the understanding of chemical reactions, bonding, and the creation of new substances from existing ones.

3. Chemistry is the central science that bridges the gap between the physical sciences (physics) and the life sciences (biology). It investigates the nature of matter and the fundamental principles governing the behavior of atoms and molecules.

CHEMICAL: 1. Chemical as a Substance: A chemical refers to a substance with a distinct molecular composition, consisting of one or more elements or compounds. These substances can undergo chemical reactions and transformations.

2. Chemical as a Process: Chemical can also describe a process involving the transformation or interaction of substances, often resulting in the creation of new compounds. This encompasses reactions such as oxidation, reduction, and synthesis.

3. Chemical as a Field of Study: Chemistry is the scientific discipline that focuses on the study of chemicals, their properties, composition, behavior, and the processes that involve them. It is a branch of science concerned with the understanding of matter at the molecular and atomic levels.

Note: Though manufactured compounds are typically included in the definition of chemicals, this is not the only use of the term.

CELL: A cell is the basic structural and functional unit of all living organisms. Some living organisms can exists only as a single cell. An average size man has about 60 to 100 trillion vells. Each cell is a small container of chemicals and water wrapped up by a thin sheet of material.

TISSUE: Tissue is a group of similar cells that work together to perform a specific function in the body. There are four primary types of tissues in the human body: epithelial, connective, muscle, and nervous tissues, each with its own distinct role and characteristics.

MUSCLE: Muscle is a contractile tissue in the human body that is responsible for various functions, including movement, support, and maintaining posture. Muscles are composed of bundles of muscle fibers that can contract and relax, generating force to move the body's bones and perform various tasks.

FAT: 1. Fat, in the context of nutrition and biology, refers to a type of organic molecule known as a lipid that is a concentrated source of energy in the form of long-chain fatty acids. Fat is an essential component of the diet and plays various roles in the body, including energy storage, insulation, and as a structural component of cell membranes.

2. Fat In biology and anatomy, fat refers to adipose tissue, which is a type of connective tissue that stores energy in the form of triglycerides. It also insulates the body and cushions organs.

3. In nutrition, fat is a macronutrient that provides essential fatty acids and serves as a source of concentrated energy. It can be found in various

foods, such as oils, nuts, and animal products, and is an important part of a balanced diet.

ORGAN: An organ is a distinct and specialized structure within an organism's body that performs a specific function or set of functions. Organs are composed of different types of tissues and are integral to the overall functioning of the organism. Examples of organs in the human body include the heart, lungs, liver, and kidneys.

GRAM: 1. A gram is a unit of weight in the metric system. One pound of gram is 454 grams.

2. Gram (g): A unit of mass in the metric system, equal to one one-thousandth of a kilogram. It is commonly used for measuring the weight of small objects or ingredients in cooking.

KILOGRAM: 1. A kilogram (kg) is the base unit of mass in the International System of Units (SI). It is defined as the mass of the International Prototype of the Kilogram (IPK), a platinum-iridium cylinder kept at the International Bureau of Weights and Measures (BIPM) in France. This definition was refined in 2019 as part of the redefinition of the SI units, linking the kilogram to fundamental constants of nature.

2. A kilogram is equal to a thousand grams. There are little more than two pounds to every kilogram.

MILLIGRAM: One thousandth of a gram is called a milligram. A gram is made up of 1,000 milligrams. A milligram is equivalent to 0.00001 grams.

CELSIUS: Celsius is a scale of temperature on which water freezes at 0 degrees (0^0) and boils at 100 degrees (100^0).

CALORIE: Calorie is a unit of measurement for energy. They are used to quantify the amount of energy that food and beverages provide when consumed. Your daily calorie intake depends on various factors such as age, gender, activity level, and weight goals.

Note: It's important to maintain a balanced calorie intake to support your overall health and well-being.

NUTRIENT: A nutrient is a substance that gives the body something that it needs to live and grow properly.

FOOD: Food is a material or substance taken into the body to provide it with nutrients it requires for energy and growth.

ELEMENT: An element, in the context of chemistry, is a substance that cannot be broken down into simpler substances by chemical means. Each element is characterized by its unique atomic number, which corresponds to the number of protons in the nucleus of its atoms.

COMPOUND: A Compound is a substance that is made of two or more elements.

BREAKDOWN: Is to separate into smaller parts.

MOLECULE: A molecule is a group of two or more atoms chemically bonded together. These atoms can be of the same or different elements, and they are the smallest units of a chemical compound that retains its chemical properties. Molecules can vary in size and complexity, from simple diatomic molecules like oxygen (O2) to large, complex molecules like DNA.

PROTEIN: Proteins are complex macromolecules composed of amino acids. They are essential biological molecules that perform a wide range of functions in living organisms. Proteins serve as structural components, enzymes, antibodies, and more, playing crucial roles in the body's growth, repair, and various biochemical processes.

ACID: An acid is a chemical substance that can donate a proton (H+) or accept an electron pair in a chemical reaction. Acids typically have a sour taste, can turn blue litmus paper red, and have a pH value less than 7 in aqueous solutions. They are an essential part of acid-base chemistry and play various roles in many chemical processes and biological systems.

AMINO ACIDS: Amino acids are very units of materials that protein is built out of.

GAS: A gas is a substance that is in an air like form. They are neither solid nor liquid.

CARBON: Carbon is fundamental to life on Earth and is the basis for organic chemistry, as it forms the backbone of many organic compounds, including carbohydrates, proteins, and nucleic acids.

HYDROGEN: Hydrogen is an odorless, colourless gas that is flammable and is the most abundant chemical element in the universe.

OXYGEN: Oxygen is a colourless, odorless chemical element and is necessary for the survival of most living things.

CARBOHYDRATE: Carbohydrate is one of the three primary macronutrients and a class of organic compounds consisting of carbon, hydrogen, and oxygen atoms. They serve as a crucial source of energy for living organisms, including humans. Carbohydrates can be found in various forms, including sugars, starches, and fibers, and they are commonly found in foods like grains, fruits, vegetables, and legumes.

DIGESTION: Digestion is the process by which your body breaks down food into smaller, absorbable components. It occurs in the digestive system and involves mechanical and chemical processes that convert complex nutrients into simpler substances, which can be absorbed and used by the body for energy and nutrition.

ENZYMES: 1. Enzymes are biological molecules, typically proteins, that act as catalysts to facilitate and accelerate chemical reactions within living organisms.

2. Enzymes are catalysts that speeds up the rate of chemical reactions.

METABOLISM: Metabolism refers to the complex set of chemical reactions that occur within an organism to maintain life. It involves the processes of breaking down substances (catabolism) to release energy and building up new molecules (anabolism) for growth, repair, and other essential functions.

ANABOLISM: Anabolism is the part of metabolism in which smaller molecules are synthesized into larger and more complex molecules. It requires energy input and is responsible for the creation of biomolecules like proteins, nucleic acids, and carbohydrates. Anabolic processes are involved in growth and tissue repair.

CATABOLISM: Catabolism is the opposite of anabolism, where larger molecules are broken down into smaller ones, releasing energy in the process. This energy is often used for various cellular activities. Catabolic processes break down molecules like carbohydrates, fats, and proteins to release energy and raw materials for anabolism.

Chapter 3

WHAT THE MAJORITY OF PEOPLE DON'T KNOW ABOUT HEALTH, NUTRITION AND FITNESS

PART TWO: HEALTH

SUPPLEMENT: A supplement is a product or substance that is intended to provide additional nutrients, vitamins, minerals, or other compounds to a person's diet. Supplements are often used to fill nutritional gaps, promote health, or address specific dietary needs. They come in various forms, such as pills, capsules, powders, and liquids.

DIETARY SUPPLEMENT: A dietary supplement is a product intended to provide nutrients that may be missing or insufficient in a person's diet. These supplements can include vitamins, minerals, herbs, amino acids, enzymes, and other substances, and are available in various forms such as pills, capsules, powders, or liquids. They are not meant to replace a balanced diet but to complement it by filling nutritional gaps or supporting specific health goals. Dietary supplements should be used with caution and under the guidance of a healthcare professional, as excessive or inappropriate use can have adverse effects.

VITAMIN: Vitamins are essential organic compounds that the human body requires in small amounts to maintain various biological functions and overall health. They play critical roles in processes like growth, metabolism, and maintaining the normal functioning of cells and tissues. There are different types of vitamins, each with specific functions and sources, such as vitamin C from citrus fruits or vitamin D from sunlight exposure.

MINERAL: A mineral is a naturally occurring, inorganic solid substance with a specific chemical composition and a crystalline structure. Minerals are the building blocks of rocks and have various physical and chemical properties that distinguish them from one another. They can be found in the Earth's crust and have been used by humans for various purposes, such as in industry and as gemstones.

HYDRATION: Hydration is the process of increasing the water content in your body, typically by drinking fluids. It helps maintain the body's water balance, supports various bodily functions, and prevents dehydration. The human body is made of 75% water.

DEHYDRATION: Dehydration is the opposite of hydration and occurs when the body loses more fluids than it takes in. This can result from inadequate fluid intake, excessive sweating, vomiting, or diarrhea, and it can lead to various health issues due to a lack of proper water levels in the body.

NERVE: A nerve is a bundle of specialized cells (neurons) that transmit signals in the form of electrical impulses between various parts of the body, allowing for communication between the brain and different organs, muscles, and tissues.

SALT: Salt, in a chemical context, refers to a compound formed when the hydrogen ions of an acid are replaced by metal ions or other cations. Common table salt, for example, is sodium chloride ($NaCl$), where sodium ions ($Na+$) replace the hydrogen ions of hydrochloric acid (HCl). Salts can have various chemical compositions and are essential in many chemical and biological processes. In everyday language, *"salt"* usually refers to common table salt, which is used as a seasoning and preservative.

PROCESSED: Processed typically refers to food or other products that have undergone various manufacturing, cooking, or preservation techniques to change their original state. These processes can include canning, freezing, drying, cooking, or adding preservatives, and they are often done to improve the shelf life, taste, or convenience of the product. However, not all processed foods are necessarily unhealthy, as some processing methods can be used to make foods safer or more nutritious. The extent and type of processing can vary widely, from minimally processed items like frozen vegetables to highly processed and heavily refined products like sugary snacks.

ORGANIC: Organic food is produced using agricultural practices that minimize synthetic chemicals and promote environmentally sustainable methods. It typically involves the use of natural fertilizers, non-synthetic pesticides, and the avoidance of genetically modified organisms (GMOs). Organic farming aims to enhance soil and ecosystem health while producing food without artificial additives or preservatives.

CHOLESTEROL: Cholesterol is a waxy, fat-like substance found in the cells of your body and in the food you eat. It is essential for building cell membranes, producing hormones, and aiding in various bodily functions. Cholesterol is transported in the bloodstream and can be categorized into "good" (HDL) and "bad" (LDL) cholesterol, with high levels of LDL cholesterol being associated with an increased risk of heart disease.

BODY MASS INDEX (BMI): Body Mass Index (BMI) is a numerical measure of a person's weight in relation to their height. It is calculated by dividing a person's weight in kilograms by the square of their height in meters. The resulting BMI value is used to classify individuals into different categories, such as underweight, normal weight, overweight, or obese, which can provide a general indication of whether a person's weight falls within a healthy range. However, it's important to note that BMI is a simplified metric and does not take into account other factors like muscle mass or distribution of weight, so it may not be a perfect measure of an individual's overall health.

PERCENTAGE: A percentage is a way of expressing a number as a fraction of 100. It is often represented by the symbol "%." For example, if you have 25%, it means you have 25 out of every 100 units or 0.25 when expressed as a decimal. Percentages are commonly used to describe proportions, ratios, or comparisons in various contexts, such as finance, statistics, and everyday calculations.

BODY FAT PERCENTAGE: Body fat percentage is a measurement that expresses the proportion of a person's total body weight that is composed of fat tissue. It is typically calculated by dividing the weight of the body fat by the total body weight and multiplying the result by 100 to express it as a percentage. This measurement is often used as an indicator of a person's overall health and fitness, as excessively high body fat percentages can be associated with various health risks.

OBESE: Obesity is a medical condition characterized by an excessive accumulation of body fat that can have negative effects on a person's health. It is typically defined by a high body mass index (BMI), which is calculated based on a person's weight and height. A BMI of 30 or higher is generally considered indicative of obesity. Obese individuals are at increased risk of various health problems, including heart disease, diabetes, and certain types of cancer.

OVERWEIGHTT: Overweight is a term used to describe a person who has a body weight that exceeds what is considered healthy or normal for their height and build. It is often determined by calculating the body mass index (BMI), with a BMI between 25 and 29.9 generally indicating overweight.

Chapter 4

WHAT THE MAJORITY OF PEOPLE DON'T KNOW ABOUT HEALTH NUTRITION AND FITNESS

PART THREE: NUTRITION

NUTRITION: 1. Nutrition is the process by which organisms obtain and use food for growth, maintenance, and energy. It involves the intake of nutrients, digestion, absorption, and utilization of these nutrients by the body to support various physiological functions.

2. Nutrition refers to the science that studies the relationship between food, nutrients, and health. It encompasses the study of the composition of foods, the dietary requirements of individuals, and how food choices can impact overall well-being.

3. Nutrition can also be defined as the sum of all processes involved in the consumption, digestion, absorption, and utilization of nutrients by the body. It's a critical aspect of maintaining good health and preventing nutritional deficiencies or excesses.

DIET: 1. Diet refers to the types and amounts of food and beverages an individual regularly consumes as part of their daily life.

2. Diet can also refer to the sum of all the food and nutrients that sustain an organism's life, whether it's a human, animal, or even a plant.

3. A diet refers to the sum of food and beverages consumed by an individual or a group. It encompasses the daily or habitual consumption of nutrients to nourish the body.

HEALTH: 1. Health is a state of overall physical, mental, and social well-being in which an individual's body and mind function optimally, free from illness, disease, or impairment. It encompasses not just the absence of illness, but also the presence of positive qualities that contribute to a person's quality of life.

2. The biomedical model of health defines it as the absence of disease and the proper functioning of the body's physiological systems. This definition primarily focuses on the physical aspects of health.

3. The World Health Organization (WHO) defines health as "a state of complete physical, mental, and social well-being and not merely the absence of disease or infirmity." This definition emphasizes that health encompasses not just the absence of illness but also the overall well-being of an individual.

HEALTHY: Simply means being in a good condition physically with good strength and energy level free from damage or illness.

2. Healthy Is a state of physical well-being, strength, and energy that is unaffected by disease or injury.

3. Healthy" typically refers to a state of well-being and balance in the physical, mental, and social aspects of a person's life. It often implies good physical health, absence of disease or illness, proper nutrition, regular exercise, and a positive mental and emotional state. However, the specific definition of "healthy" can vary depending on context and individual circumstances.

NOURISH: 1. Nourish means to supply the body with essential nutrients and sustenance, such as food and water, to support its growth and well-being.

2. Nourish is to provide something with substances needed to live, grow and stay healthy.

SUGAR: Sugar is a type of sweet-tasting carbohydrates that can be found in a variety of foods, including honey, fruits, and plants.

SUCROSE: Sucrose is a disaccharide sugar composed of two simpler sugars, glucose and fructose, linked together. It is commonly known as table sugar and is often used as a sweetener in various food and beverage products. Sucrose is naturally found in many plants, especially in sugar cane and sugar beets, and is an essential source of energy in the human diet.

GLUCOSE: Glucose is a simple sugar that is an important source of energy in living things.

2. Glucose is a simple sugar, also known as a monosaccharide, that serves as a primary source of energy for living organisms. It is a

carbohydrate and is commonly found in various foods, especially in carbohydrates like bread, rice, and fruits. Glucose is essential for cellular respiration, where it is metabolized to produce ATP (adenosine triphosphate), the primary energy currency of cells. It has the chemical formula $C_6H_{12}O_6$.

GLYCOGEN: Glycogen is a complex carbohydrate that serves as a form of energy storage in animals, including humans. It is primarily found in the liver and muscles and can be quickly broken down into glucose when the body needs energy. Glycogen plays a crucial role in regulating blood sugar levels and providing a readily available source of energy during periods of high physical activity or between meals.

BLOOD SUGAR: Is the amount of glucose in the blood. Blood carries glucose, which is sent to cells where it is broken down to provide energy that can be consumed or stored.

SIMPLE CARBOHYDRATE: Simple carbohydrates, often referred to as "simple sugars," are composed of one or two sugar units (monosaccharides or disaccharides). Common examples include glucose, fructose, and sucrose (table sugar). These sugars are quickly digested and can cause rapid spikes in blood sugar levels.

COMPLEX CARBOHYDRATE: Complex carbohydrates, on the other hand, are composed of long chains of sugar units (polysaccharides) and take longer to break down during digestion. Common sources of complex carbohydrates include foods like whole grains, starchy vegetables, and legumes. They provide a more sustained release of energy and are often a healthier choice due to their fiber and nutrient content.

STARCH: Starch is a complex carbohydrate consisting of long chains of glucose molecules linked together. It serves as a primary storage form of energy in plants and can be found in various plant-based foods like potatoes, rice, wheat, and corn. Starch can be broken down into simpler sugars through digestion and serves as a significant source of energy for humans and animals.

HORMONES: Hormones are chemical messengers produced by glands in the endocrine system that regulate various physiological processes in the body. They travel through the bloodstream to target cells or organs, where they influence functions such as growth, metabolism, reproduction, and mood.

INSULIN: Insulin is a hormone produced by the pancreas that plays a crucial role in regulating blood sugar (glucose) levels in the body. It allows cells to take in and use glucose for energy, which helps lower blood sugar levels. Insulin also helps store excess glucose in the liver for later use. Insufficient insulin production or resistance to its effects can lead to high blood sugar levels, which is a characteristic of diabetes.

INDEX: And index is a system of listing informations in order to allow one to easily compare them to other informations.

GLYCEMIC INDEX: The glycemic index (GI) is a measure of how quickly carbohydrates in a food raise blood sugar levels after consumption. Foods with a high GI are rapidly digested and cause a quick spike in blood sugar, while foods with a low GI are digested more slowly and result in a more gradual and steady increase in blood sugar levels. The scale typically ranges from 0 to 100, with higher values indicating a higher impact on blood sugar. Low-GI foods are often considered healthier choices for managing blood sugar and providing sustained energy.

GRAIN: Grains are small, hard, edible seeds that are the harvested fruits of various cereal crops. They are a significant source of carbohydrates, providing energy in the form of starch. Common grains include wheat, rice, corn, oats, barley, and rye. Grains are a staple in many diets around the world and serve as the basis for various food products such as bread, pasta, and cereal.

WHOLE GRAIN: Whole grains are grains that contain all parts of the original kernel, including the bran, germ, and endosperm. This means they retain more of their natural nutrients, fiber, and flavor compared to refined grains, where the bran and germ are removed during processing. Common whole grains include wheat, oats, rice, barley, and quinoa, among others. Consuming whole grains is associated with various health benefits due to their higher nutritional content.

WHEAT: Wheat is a cereal grain that is widely cultivated and used for its edible seeds. It is a staple food in many parts of the world and is a primary ingredient in various food products, including bread, pasta, and cereal. Wheat comes in different varieties, including common wheat (Triticum aestivum) and durum wheat (Triticum durum), each with distinct characteristics and uses.

WHITE BREAD: White bread is a type of bread made from wheat flour that has had the bran and germ removed, leaving only the starchy endosperm. It is typically softer and lighter in color compared to whole wheat or whole grain bread. White bread is a common staple in many diets and is known for its mild flavor and soft texture.

FIBER: Fiber, refers to the indigestible portion of plant-based foods. It is a type of carbohydrate that cannot be broken down by the human digestive system. Dietary fiber comes in two main forms: soluble and insoluble, and it plays a crucial role in promoting digestive health, regulating blood sugar levels, and supporting heart health. It is found in foods like fruits, vegetables, whole grains, and legumes.

FATTY ACIDS: Fatty acids are organic molecules that serve as important building blocks of lipids, such as fats and oils.

ESSENTIAL FATTY ACIDS: Essential fatty acids are types of fats that the human body cannot produce on its own and must obtain through dietary sources. These fats are necessary for various physiological functions and are classified into two main types: omega-3 fatty acids and omega-6 fatty acids. They play a crucial role in maintaining healthy cell membranes, brain function, and overall well-being. Common food sources of essential fatty acids include fish, nuts, seeds, and vegetable oils.

FATS: Fats, also known as lipids, are organic molecules that are an essential part of a healthy diet. They are a concentrated source of energy and serve various critical functions in the body, including insulating and protecting organs, maintaining cell membranes, and aiding in the absorption of fat-soluble vitamins. Fats are composed of fatty acids and come in various types, such as saturated fats, unsaturated fats (monounsaturated and polyunsaturated), and trans fats, each with different effects on health.

OIL: Oil is a viscous liquid composed of hydrocarbons, typically derived from petroleum or other sources. It is a crucial source of energy, used in various industries, and can also refer to edible oils used in cooking, such as vegetable oil or olive oil.

Chapter 5

THE ACTUAL SCIENCE OF GROWTH IN MUSCLE

The actual science of muscle growth, also known as muscle hypertrophy, is a fascinating field of study within exercise physiology and biology. It involves understanding the intricate processes that occur at the cellular and molecular levels as our muscles adapt to various forms of resistance training. Muscle growth is not merely a result of lifting weights; it's a complex biological phenomenon influenced by genetics, nutrition, hormonal factors, and training methods.

At its core, muscle growth is driven by the hypertrophy of individual muscle fibers. When subjected to mechanical tension, muscle fibers undergo a series of events that lead to their enlargement. This process typically involves damage to muscle fibers, followed by repair and growth. Key factors that influence muscle growth include protein synthesis, satellite cell activation, and the regulation of anabolic hormones like testosterone and growth hormone.

Understanding the science of muscle growth is crucial for athletes, bodybuilders, and fitness enthusiasts, as it allows for more effective training and nutrition strategies. This science-based approach helps individuals optimize their workouts, recovery, and dietary choices to achieve their desired muscle-building goals. Whether you're looking to gain strength, improve your physique, or enhance your athletic performance, delving into the actual science of muscle growth can provide valuable insights to help you reach your objectives.

The science of muscle growth, also known as muscle hypertrophy, involves several key principles:

THE FIRST PRINCIPLE OF MUSCLE GROWTH:
<u>Muscle Fiber Recruitment</u>

Muscle fiber recruitment is a crucial concept in bodybuilding and resistance training. It refers to the process by which your body activates different types of muscle fibers to generate force and perform a specific movement or exercise. There are two primary types of muscle fibers:

1. **Slow-Twitch (Type I) Muscle Fibers**: These fibers are more endurance-oriented and are recruited for low-intensity, long-duration activities. They have a high resistance to fatigue and are responsible for maintaining posture and performing activities like jogging or cycling.

2. **Fast-Twitch (Type II) Muscle Fibers**: These fibers are geared towards generating rapid, intense bursts of power and are further divided into Type IIa and Type IIb fibers. Type IIa fibers have a mix of endurance and strength characteristics, while Type IIb fibers are primarily for short, high-intensity efforts.

In bodybuilding, the goal is often to target and stimulate as many muscle fibers as possible to promote muscle growth and strength. Here's how muscle fiber recruitment works in this context:

- **Warm-Up**: The initial phase of your workout involves using lighter weights and exercises to warm up your muscles and activate a small number of muscle fibers.

- **Progressive Resistance**: As you increase the weight or resistance, your body recruits more muscle fibers to meet the demand. Initially, slow-twitch fibers are engaged, but as the intensity rises, fast-twitch fibers come into play.

- **Repetition Range**: The number of repetitions you perform and the weight you lift affect which muscle fibers are recruited. Higher repetitions with lower weights primarily engage slow-twitch fibers, while lower repetitions with heavier weights target fast-twitch fibers.

- **Varied Exercises**: Bodybuilders often incorporate a variety of exercises to target different muscle groups and stimulate a broad range of muscle fibers. Compound movements like squats and deadlifts engage multiple muscle groups and both slow and fast-twitch fibers.

- **Fatigue**: As you continue your workout, muscle fibers become fatigued. When slow-twitch fibers tire, your body recruits fast-twitch fibers to help maintain force production.

When you engage in resistance training (e.g., weightlifting), your body recruits muscle fibers to overcome the resistance. Initially, it activates smaller, slow-twitch muscle fibers, and as the load or intensity increases, it recruits larger, fast-twitch muscle fibers.

It's essential to design your training program with an understanding of muscle fiber recruitment to achieve balanced muscle development and optimize your bodybuilding results. Tailoring your workouts to target both slow and fast-twitch muscle fibers can lead to more significant gains in muscle size and strength.

THE SECOND PRINCIPLE OF MUSCLE GROWTH: Progressive Overload

Progressive overload is a fundamental principle in bodybuilding and strength training. It involves gradually increasing the demands placed on your muscles over time to promote muscle growth and strength gains. This can be achieved by:

1. **Increasing Weight**: Gradually lifting heavier weights as your strength improves. This challenges your muscles to adapt and grow.

2. **Increasing Reps and Sets**: Adding more repetitions or sets to your workouts over time can increase the workload on your muscles.

3. Increasing Intensity: You can intensify your workouts by reducing rest times between sets or performing exercises with stricter form.

4. Varying Exercises: Switching to different exercises or variations can target muscles from different angles, preventing plateaus.

To stimulate muscle growth, you need to progressively increase the resistance or workload over time. This forces your muscles to adapt and grow stronger.

The idea is to continually push your limits to stimulate muscle adaptation. Progressive overload is key to achieving long-term gains in muscle size and strength.

THE THIRD PRINCIPLE OF MUSCLE GROWTH:
<u>Muscle Damage and Repair</u>

Muscle damage and repair are essential processes in bodybuilding and muscle growth. Here's a simplified explanation:

- **Muscle Damage**: During intense workouts, especially when you lift heavy weights or perform challenging exercises, you cause microtears in your muscle fibers. This is often referred to as muscle damage. It's a natural and necessary part of the muscle-building process.

- **Inflammation**: Muscle damage triggers an inflammatory response in your body. Inflammation is the initial step in the repair process. It helps remove damaged tissue and initiate the healing process.

- **Protein Synthesis:** After muscle damage, your body starts to repair and rebuild the damaged muscle fibers. This is where protein synthesis comes into play. Your body utilizes dietary protein to create new muscle protein, making the repaired muscle fibers thicker and stronger.

- **Muscle Hypertrophy**: Over time, as you continue to challenge your muscles and provide them with the necessary nutrients (especially protein), they adapt and grow in size and strength. This process is called muscle hypertrophy.

- **Rest and Nutrition**: To optimize muscle repair and growth, it's crucial to allow your muscles adequate rest between workouts. Additionally, a balanced diet with sufficient protein, carbohydrates, and fats is essential to support muscle repair and overall recovery.

Resistance training causes microscopic damage to muscle fibers. The body responds by repairing and overcompensating, leading to muscle growth.

Remember that muscle damage and repair are continuous processes in bodybuilding. Providing your body with the right stimulus through workouts, proper nutrition, and adequate rest is key to maximizing your muscle growth and strength gains.

THE FOURTH PRINCIPLE OF MUSCLE GROWTH: <u>Nutrition</u>

I won't linger on or say too much about nutrition because we've been discussing it from the beginning of this book.

Adequate nutrition is essential for muscle growth. Protein intake, in particular, is crucial because it provides the building blocks (amino acids) necessary for muscle repair and growth.

THE FIFTH PRINCIPLE OF MUSCLE GROWTH: <u>Rest and Recovery</u>

Rest and Recovery: Muscles need time to recover and grow. Proper sleep, rest between workouts, and managing stress are important for this process.

Rest and recovery are crucial components of bodybuilding workouts. Here's an explanation of their significance:

- **Rest Days**: These are scheduled breaks in your training routine where you give your muscles time to recuperate. During intense workouts, muscle fibers undergo tiny tears, and rest days allow them to heal and grow stronger. Rest days can vary depending on your training program but are typically taken between weightlifting sessions for the same muscle group. They help prevent overtraining, reduce the risk of injury, and promote muscle growth.

- **Recovery**: Recovery encompasses various strategies to enhance the healing and adaptation of muscles. This includes proper nutrition, hydration, and sleep. Consuming adequate protein and nutrients is essential for muscle repair and growth. Staying hydrated is crucial for overall well-being and muscle function. Sleep is when the body releases growth hormone and repairs muscle tissue, so quality rest is vital.

- **Active Recovery**: Some individuals incorporate light, low-intensity activities like walking, swimming, or yoga on rest days. This can help improve blood circulation, reduce muscle soreness, and aid in recovery without putting excessive strain on the muscles.

- **Periodization**: Effective bodybuilding programs often use periodization, which involves planned variations in training intensity and volume. This allows for adequate recovery between more intense phases of training and helps prevent plateaus in muscle growth.

- **Listen to Your Body**: Pay attention to your body's signals. If you're feeling fatigued, sore, or notice a drop in performance, it may be a sign that you need more rest. Pushing too hard without sufficient recovery can lead to burnout and increased risk of injuries.

In bodybuilding, progress is not just about lifting heavier weights; it's also about giving your body the time and resources it needs to repair and grow. Balancing training with proper rest and recovery is essential for achieving your fitness goals while staying healthy and injury-free.

THE SIXTH PRINCIPLE OF MUSCLE GROWTH:
<u>Hormones</u>

Hormones: Hormones like testosterone, growth hormone, and insulin-like growth factor play a role in muscle growth. However, genetics, age, and sex also influence hormone levels and their impact on muscle growth.

Hormones play a crucial role in bodybuilding workouts by influencing muscle growth, energy levels, and overall performance. Here are some key hormones and their roles in this context:

- **Testosterone**: Testosterone is a primary hormone for muscle growth. It increases protein synthesis, enhances muscle recovery, and boosts strength. Bodybuilders often seek to optimize their testosterone levels through proper nutrition, resistance training, and adequate sleep.

- **Growth Hormone (GH):** GH stimulates the growth and repair of tissues, including muscles. It helps increase muscle mass and reduce fat. Intense workouts and deep sleep can trigger the release of GH.

- **Insulin**: Insulin plays a role in nutrient uptake by cells. Post-workout, it helps shuttle glucose and amino acids into muscles, aiding recovery and growth. Controlling insulin levels through diet is essential for bodybuilders.

- **Cortisol**: Cortisol is a stress hormone that can break down muscle tissue when present in excess. Managing stress and avoiding overtraining is crucial to keep cortisol levels in check.

- **Epinephrine and Norepinephrine**: These "fight or flight" hormones provide an energy boost during intense workouts. They increase heart rate, blood flow, and focus, helping bodybuilders push through challenging sessions.

- **Thyroid Hormones**: Thyroid hormones influence metabolism and energy expenditure. Proper thyroid function is vital for maintaining an optimal body composition and energy levels.

- **Estrogen and Progesterone (in women):** These hormones affect muscle growth, fat storage, and water retention. Bodybuilders may need to manage these hormones to optimize their physique.

- **Leptin and Ghrelin**: These hormones regulate appetite and hunger. Managing them can be important for maintaining a bodybuilder's desired body fat percentage.

Overall, understanding and balancing these hormones through training, nutrition, and lifestyle choices are essential for bodybuilders looking to achieve their goals of muscle hypertrophy, reduced body fat, and improved performance. It's important to note that manipulating hormones should always be done under the guidance of a healthcare professional to ensure safety and effectiveness.

THE SEVENTH PRINCIPLE OF MUSCLE GROWTH: Volume and Frequency

Volume and Frequency: The volume (sets and reps) and frequency (how often you train a muscle group) of your workouts are important factors. Different training programs can be tailored to specific goals, whether it's strength, hypertrophy, or endurance.

Volume and frequency are two essential concepts in bodybuilding workouts that play a significant role in achieving muscle growth and strength. Here's a brief explanation of each:

Volume:
- Volume refers to the total amount of work you perform in a workout, typically measured by the total number of sets and repetitions you complete.
- In bodybuilding, higher volume workouts involve more sets and repetitions. This can lead to greater muscle hypertrophy (growth) as it creates more time under tension for the muscles.
- Common volume-related terms include "total volume load," which is the weight lifted in a session multiplied by the number of sets and reps.

Frequency:
- Frequency relates to how often you perform a particular workout or train a specific muscle group.
- Higher frequency means you work out a muscle group or perform a particular exercise more frequently throughout the week.
- Adequate frequency is crucial for stimulating muscle growth and ensuring that each muscle group receives sufficient attention and recovery.

Balancing volume and frequency in your bodybuilding workouts is essential. Here are some key points to consider:

- Higher volume workouts can be effective for muscle growth but may require longer recovery periods between sessions.
- Frequency can be adjusted based on your goals and preferences. Some bodybuilders use a split routine (working different muscle groups on different days) to increase frequency.
- Overtraining can occur if you push volume and frequency to extremes, leading to diminishing returns and increased risk of injury.

- Periodization, which involves adjusting volume and frequency over time, can help prevent plateaus and optimize muscle gains.

Ultimately, the right balance of volume and frequency in your bodybuilding workouts depends on your individual goals, experience, and recovery capacity. It's advisable to consult with a fitness professional or trainer to design a workout plan tailored to your specific needs.

THE EIGHTH PRINCIPLE OF MUSCLE GROWTH: Muscle Protein Synthesis

Muscle Protein Synthesis: Muscle growth is driven by the process of muscle protein synthesis, where new proteins are built in muscle fibers. This process is influenced by factors like exercise, nutrition, and hormone levels.

Muscle Protein Synthesis (MPS) is a key process in bodybuilding and muscle growth. It refers to the creation of new muscle protein fibers within your muscle cells, leading to muscle hypertrophy (growth). Here's a simplified explanation of how it works:

1. **Muscle Damage**: During intense weightlifting or resistance training, your muscles experience micro-tears.

2. **Recovery Phase**: After your workout, your body initiates the repair and recovery process. This is when MPS is crucial.

3. **Protein Intake**: Consuming an adequate amount of protein, especially essential amino acids, is essential. Amino acids are the building blocks of protein.

4. **Protein Synthesis**: MPS is the process where amino acids are assembled into new muscle proteins. This occurs primarily in response to the stress placed on the muscles during exercise and the availability of amino acids from your diet.

5. **Anabolism**: The newly synthesized proteins are added to your muscle cells, making them bigger and stronger. This is the anabolic phase of muscle growth.

Factors that influence MPS in bodybuilding include the intensity of your workouts, the timing of protein consumption, and your overall nutrition and recovery strategies. Maximizing MPS through proper training and nutrition is essential for muscle development and achieving bodybuilding goals.

THE NINTH PRINCIPLE OF MUSCLE GROWTH:
Genetics

Genetics: Genetics can significantly influence how your body responds to resistance training and the rate at which you can gain muscle mass.

Genetics plays a significant role in bodybuilding workouts in several ways:

- **Muscle Fiber Type**: Genetics determine your muscle fiber composition, which can affect your ability to build muscle. Some people have a higher proportion of fast-twitch muscle fibers, which are better suited for explosive strength and muscle growth, while others have more slow-twitch fibers, which are better for endurance activities. This can influence how quickly and how much muscle you can develop.

- **Muscle Insertions**: Genetics also influence the placement of muscle insertions, which can affect the shape and appearance of your muscles. Some individuals may naturally have more favorable muscle insertion points for certain exercises, which can lead to better results in those specific muscle groups.

- **Metabolism**: Your metabolic rate is influenced by genetics. Some people naturally have a faster metabolism, making it easier for them to stay lean and build muscle, while others may have a slower metabolism, which can make it more challenging to achieve desired results.

- **Hormonal Factors**: Hormones like testosterone and growth hormone play a crucial role in muscle growth. Genetics can influence your baseline hormone levels, which can impact your body's ability to build muscle.

- **Recovery and Adaptation**: Genetic factors can affect how quickly your body recovers from workouts and adapts to training stimuli. Some individuals may recover faster and adapt more efficiently to exercise, leading to better gains in muscle mass.

- **Injury Susceptibility**: Genetics can also influence your susceptibility to injuries. Some people may have a genetic predisposition to certain injuries, which can affect their training consistency and progress.

While genetics do play a significant role in bodybuilding, it's important to note that hard work, proper nutrition, and consistent training can still lead to substantial improvements, regardless of your genetic predispositions. Tailoring your workouts and nutrition to your individual needs and goals is key to maximizing your bodybuilding potential.

THE TENTH PRINCIPLE OF MUSCLE GROWTH:
<u>Consistency</u>

Consistency: Consistency in training and nutrition is key. Muscle growth is a gradual process that requires dedication over time.

Consistency in bodybuilding workouts refers to the regular and reliable adherence to a structured training program over an extended period of time. It involves consistently following a workout schedule, maintaining proper form and technique, and staying committed to your fitness goals. In bodybuilding, consistency is crucial for several reasons:

- **Muscle Growth**: Consistently training specific muscle groups allows for gradual muscle hypertrophy. Regular workouts stimulate muscle fibers to grow and adapt to the resistance, resulting in increased muscle size and strength.

- **Progress Tracking**: Consistency enables you to track your progress more accurately. By regularly performing the same exercises and tracking your performance, you can assess whether you are making gains or need to adjust your training program.

- **Skill Development**: Proper form and technique are essential in bodybuilding to prevent injury and maximize muscle engagement. Consistent training helps you develop and maintain these skills over time.

- **Habit Formation**: Consistency helps form good exercise habits. When you make workouts a regular part of your routine, they become easier to stick to, increasing the likelihood of long-term success.

- **Plateau Avoidance**: Continuous variation and progression in your workouts are essential for avoiding plateaus, where your body adapts to your routine and stops making progress. Consistency helps you make systematic changes to your training program to keep seeing results.

- **Injury Prevention**: Regular training can help condition and strengthen your muscles and joints, reducing the risk of injury that may occur with sporadic or inconsistent workouts.

In summary, consistency is a fundamental principle in bodybuilding that contributes to muscle growth, progress tracking, skill development, habit formation, plateau avoidance, and injury prevention. To achieve your bodybuilding goals, it's crucial to maintain a consistent and disciplined workout regimen.

Remember that individual responses to training and nutrition can vary, and what works best for one person may not be the same for another. It's important to tailor your approach to your specific goals and body's response to training. Consulting with a fitness professional or a registered dietitian can help you create an effective plan for muscle growth based on your unique needs and goals.

Chapter 6

THE 10 BIGGEST MUSCLE BUILDING MYTHS & MISTAKES

If you watch folks lifting weights at the gym, nine out of ten of them are not doing it right. To perform their workout routines in the morning, I would frequently not even bother getting out of bed.

Usually, people are adhering to programs that they obtained from friends or trainers, or they may have found them online or in periodicals. They are unable to break through or are making slow, obstinate progress.

The majority of people also make a number of additional muscle-robbing errors when it comes to their diet, including eating too much, too little, and not obtaining the proper kinds and amounts of macronutrients.

So, since developing lean muscle will be crucial to creating the physique of your dreams, allow me to take a time to address the top 10 myths (misconceptions) and mistakes (errors) regarding this process.

It is highly likely that you have fallen prey to one or more of these fallacies in the past. If you haven't succumbed, it's likely because you are a newbie, which is actually a huge advantage since you get to start off correctly.

MYTH AND MISTAKE 1
Spot Reduction

Myth - You can burn fat from specific areas by targeting them with exercises.

Mistake - Fat loss occurs uniformly throughout the body, not just in the area you work.

MYTH AND MISTAKE 2
High Reps for Cutting

Myth - High-repetition, low-weight workouts are best for cutting.

Mistake - Muscle growth is primarily achieved through progressive overload with heavy weights, even when cutting.

MYTH AND MISTAKE 3
No Pain, No Gain

Myth - You must feel extreme muscle soreness to build muscle.

Mistake - Muscle soreness isn't a direct indicator of muscle growth, and overtraining can lead to injury.

MYTH AND MISTAKE 4
Excessive Protein

Myth - You need huge amounts of protein to build muscle.

Mistake - While protein is essential, excessive consumption won't lead to more muscle growth. A balanced diet is key.

MYTHS AND MISTAKE 5
Ignoring Compound Exercises

Myth - Isolating muscles with single-joint exercises is best.

Mistake - Compound exercises like squats, deadlifts, and bench presses are more effective for overall muscle development.

MYTHS AND MISTAKE 6
Overtraining

Myth - The more you work out, the more muscle you'll build.

Mistake - Rest and recovery are crucial. Overtraining can hinder muscle growth and lead to injury.

MYTHS AND MISTAKE 7
Inconsistent Training

Myth - Inconsistency in your workout routine yields the best results.

Mistake - Consistency and a well-structured plan are vital for muscle growth.

MYTHS AND MISTAKE 8
Supplement Dependency

Myth - You need a ton of supplements for muscle growth.

Mistake - Whole foods should be your primary source of nutrition. Supplements should complement, not replace, a balanced diet.

MYTHS AND MISTAKE 9
Neglecting Cardio

Myth - Cardio hinders muscle gains.

Mistake - Cardio can aid in overall health, and moderate cardio can be incorporated into a muscle-building program without significant interference.

MYTHS AND MISTAKE 10
Lack of Sleep

Myth - Sleep isn't crucial for muscle growth.

Mistake - Quality sleep is essential for recovery and muscle repair. Inadequate sleep can hinder your progress.

Remember that individual factors, such as genetics, play a role in how your body responds to training and nutrition. It's important to tailor your approach to your specific goals and needs.

<h1 align="center">Chapter 7</h1>

THE TOP 5 MYTHS & MISTAKES REGARDING FAT LOSS

I aim to dispel the five most widespread myths and mistakes or misconceptions and errors about burning fat or fat reduction in this chapter. These misconceptions have crept into our minds, just like the ones about developing muscle, through magazines, advertisements, trainers, friends, and other sources. Let's debunk the myth that they can prevent you from achieving the toned figure you want once and for all.

When it comes to achieving a healthy and sustainable fat loss, there is a sea of information out there, some of it accurate and some not. In this exploration, we will unravel the top 5 myths and mistakes that often misguide individuals on their journey to shedding excess body fat. By dispelling these misconceptions and understanding the common errors, you can better navigate the path to achieving your fat loss goals, ensuring a more effective and scientifically informed approach. So, let's dive in and uncover the truths behind fat loss while debunking the myths and pitfalls that may be hindering your progress.

<h3 align="center">MYTH & MISTAKE 1:
Spot Reduction</h3>

Myth - You can lose fat from a specific area by targeting exercises.

Mistake - Focusing solely on exercises for one area won't reduce fat there. Fat loss is generally overall, not spot-specific.

Spot reduction is the mistaken belief that you can target fat loss from a specific area of your body by exercising that particular area. It's a myth because when you lose fat, it happens throughout your body, not just in the areas you're exercising. The body decides where it stores and removes fat based on genetic and hormonal factors, and spot reduction doesn't change that.

MYTH & MISTAKE 2:
Extreme Dieting

Myth - Crash diets and severe calorie restriction lead to sustainable fat loss.

Mistake - Extreme diets can be harmful and often lead to muscle loss, metabolic slowdown, and rebound weight gain.

Extreme dieting is often considered a myth because it promotes unrealistic and unsustainable approaches to weight loss. People may resort to severe calorie restriction, extreme food restrictions, or fad diets that promise quick results. However, these methods can be harmful, as they often lead to nutrient deficiencies, muscle loss, and can negatively impact metabolism. Sustainable and balanced dietary changes are generally more effective for long-term health and weight management.

MYTH & MISTAKE 3:
Cardio is King

Myth - Cardio is the best and only way to burn fat.

Mistake - While cardio is important, neglecting strength training and a balanced diet can hinder fat loss and muscle preservation.

Cardio is King is a myth in the context of bodybuilding because it suggests that cardiovascular exercise is the most important component of building a muscular physique. In reality, while cardio has its benefits for overall health and fat loss, it's not the primary focus for bodybuilders. Resistance training and proper nutrition are the key elements in bodybuilding, as they help to build and maintain muscle mass.

MYTH & MISTAKE 4:
Zero Fat Diet

Myth - Cutting out all fats from your diet is the way to lose fat.

Mistake - Healthy fats are essential for various bodily functions, and a balanced intake is crucial for overall health and effective fat loss.

Zero fat diets are often considered a myth because fat is an essential nutrient required for various bodily functions. Completely eliminating fat from your diet can lead to nutrient deficiencies, affect hormone production, and hinder the absorption of fat-soluble vitamins (A, D, E, and K). Instead of avoiding all fats, it's better to focus on consuming healthy fats in moderation.

MYTH & MISTAKE 5:
No Cheat Days

Myth - Avoiding all indulgent foods is necessary for fat loss.

Mistake - Occasional treats are acceptable and can help maintain a sustainable and enjoyable diet. Restricting too much can lead to cravings and binging.

The idea of "no cheat days" is a common misconception in fitness and nutrition. It suggests that one should never indulge in their favorite, less healthy foods. In reality, cheat days or occasional treats can be a part of a balanced lifestyle. Moderation is key, and rigidly avoiding indulgences can lead to an unsustainable and potentially unhealthy approach to dieting. It's important to enjoy treats in moderation while maintaining a generally healthy eating pattern.

Remember, fat loss is a complex process that involves a balanced diet, regular physical activity, and patience. It's essential to approach it with a well-rounded and sustainable plan.

Chapter 8

THE ACTUAL SCIENCE OF HEALTHY FAT LOSS

Before we get into the laws of fat loss, let me explain how your body perceives fat versus muscle. Your body perceives fat as anasset, and muscle as salability. Why?

Because thousands of years ago, when our ancestors roamed the wild, they occasionally traveled for days without food, and their bodies survived off fat stores. Eventually, starving, they would kill an animal and feast, and their bodies learned to prepare for the next bout of starvation by storing fat. Having fat was literally a matter of life and death.

This genetic programming is still present in us, ready to be put to use. If you starve your body, it will burn fat to stay alive, but it will also slow down its metabolism to conserve energy, becoming fully prepared to store fat once you start giving it larger quantities of food.

The perception of muscle is different because it requires energy to maintain. Although the precise amounts of calories required to maintain muscle are debatable, your body uses more energy to maintain a pound of muscle than it does to carry fat because it knows that maintaining a healthy weight requires calories that it may or may not get.

What does this mean for fat loss? Well, it means that you have to convince your body that there is no reason for it to store excess fat and, in essence, to climb to the desired level. The same is true for muscle building: If you don't give your body the ideal conditions for muscle growth (appropriate training, nutrition, and rest), your body will be inclined to simply not grow muscle.

Alright, let's explore the fundamental principles of fat loss.

Healthy fat loss is a complex process that involves various aspects of science, including nutrition, physiology, and psychology. Here are some key scientific principles for achieving healthy fat loss:

FIRST PRINCIPLE OF FAT LOSS:
<u>Caloric Balance</u>

Fat loss fundamentally relies on creating a caloric deficit, where you consume fewer calories than you burn. This is achieved through a combination of reducing calorie intake and increasing physical activity.

Caloric balance is a fundamental principle in bodybuilding workouts and nutrition. It refers to the relationship between the number of calories you consume through your diet and the number of calories you burn through physical activity and daily metabolic processes. In the context of bodybuilding, caloric balance plays a crucial role in achieving specific goals:

- **Caloric Surplus**: To build muscle, bodybuilders often aim for a caloric surplus. This means consuming more calories than they burn, providing the extra energy required for muscle growth. The surplus helps supply the necessary nutrients and energy for the body to repair and build new muscle tissue.

- **Caloric Deficit**: When bodybuilders want to reduce body fat and achieve a leaner physique, they may enter a caloric deficit. This involves consuming fewer calories than they burn, forcing the body to use stored fat for energy. This helps reveal the muscle definition they've worked to build.

- **Maintenance Calories**: To maintain their current physique, bodybuilders aim for a balance between calorie intake and expenditure. This allows them to preserve their muscle mass and body composition.

- **Macronutrient Composition**: Beyond calorie balance, the quality of the calories consumed is essential. Bodybuilders often pay attention to their macronutrient intake, emphasizing protein for muscle repair and growth, while also managing carbohydrates and fats to meet their energy and nutritional needs.

- **Meal Timing**: Timing meals and nutrient intake around workouts is also a key part of caloric balance. Pre-workout and post-workout nutrition can influence muscle recovery and growth.

- **Adaptation**: Bodybuilders need to be aware of the body's ability to adapt. Over time, metabolic rate and calorie requirements may change, so they may need to adjust their caloric intake to continue making progress.

Overall, understanding and managing caloric balance is critical for bodybuilders to meet their specific goals, whether it's gaining muscle, losing body fat, or maintaining their physique. It requires a combination of proper nutrition, exercise, and monitoring to achieve desired results.

SECOND PRINCIPLE OF FAT LOSS:
Macronutrient Balance

A balanced diet is crucial. Focus on getting the right proportions of carbohydrates, proteins, and healthy fats. Protein can help preserve muscle mass during fat loss.

In the context of bodybuilding workouts, achieving a balance of macronutrients is crucial for optimizing muscle growth and overall performance. Macronutrients are the three primary components of your diet: protein, carbohydrates, and fats. Here's how macronutrient balance applies to bodybuilding:

- **Protein**: Protein is essential for muscle repair and growth. Bodybuilders typically need a higher protein intake to support muscle recovery and development. Aim for around 1.2 to 2.2 grams of protein per kilogram of body weight per day.

- **Carbohydrates**: Carbohydrates provide energy for your workouts and help replenish glycogen stores in your muscles. They are crucial for sustaining intense training sessions. Ensure you consume an adequate amount of complex carbohydrates like whole grains, fruits, and vegetables.

- **Fats**: Healthy fats are necessary for hormone production and overall health. While bodybuilders often focus on protein and carbs, it's essential not to neglect fats. Include sources of unsaturated fats such as avocados, nuts, and olive oil in your diet.

The specific balance of macronutrients may vary depending on individual goals and body types. Some bodybuilders follow a macronutrient ratio like 40% carbohydrates, 30% protein, and 30% fats, but these ratios can be adjusted to meet your unique needs.

Remember, consistency and tracking your nutrition are key in achieving your bodybuilding goals. It's often advisable to consult with a nutritionist or dietitian to create a customized plan that aligns with your training and body composition objectives.

THIRD PRINCIPLE OF FAT LOSS:
<u>Energy Expenditure</u>

Your basal metabolic rate (BMR) and physical activity level determine how many calories you burn daily. Increasing your BMR through muscle mass and staying active can aid fat loss.

Energy expenditure plays a crucial role in fat loss within the context of bodybuilding workouts. The principle of energy expenditure is based on the concept that in order to lose fat, you must create a calorie deficit, where you burn more calories than you consume. Here's how it applies to bodybuilding workouts:

- **Caloric Deficit**: To lose fat, you need to consume fewer calories than your body expends. Bodybuilding workouts, which often involve resistance training, can help increase your daily energy expenditure. This happens through the energy needed to lift weights, perform exercises, and repair muscle tissue after the workout.

- **Metabolic Rate**: Bodybuilding can help increase your basal metabolic rate (BMR). Muscle tissue burns more calories at rest than fat tissue, so as you build muscle, your BMR increases, leading to greater energy expenditure even when you're not working out.

- **High-Intensity Workouts**: Many bodybuilding workouts incorporate high-intensity interval training (HIIT) or circuit training, which can boost calorie burn during the workout and even post-workout due to the afterburn effect.

- **Long-Term Impact**: Regular bodybuilding workouts help you maintain lean muscle mass. This is vital for fat loss because muscle tissue is metabolically active and burns more calories than fat. So, maintaining and building muscle contributes to ongoing energy expenditure.

- **Nutrition**: To optimize fat loss, it's important to pair bodybuilding workouts with a balanced, calorie-controlled diet. This ensures that you maintain a caloric deficit, helping you tap into stored fat for energy.

- **Consistency**: Consistency in both workouts and nutrition is key. Sustainable fat loss requires a sustained calorie deficit, which is best achieved through regular exercise and a healthy diet.

In summary, energy expenditure is a fundamental principle in fat loss for bodybuilders. Through bodybuilding workouts, you can increase your energy expenditure, improve your metabolic rate, and build muscle, all of which contribute to creating a caloric deficit and ultimately shedding body fat. However, it's essential to combine these workouts with a well-balanced diet and maintain consistency for long-term success.

FOURTH PRINCIPLE OF FAT LOSS:
Portion Control

Controlling portion sizes helps regulate calorie intake. Eating mindfully and avoiding overeating are important aspects of fat loss.

Portion control is a fundamental principle of fat loss that involves managing the amount of food you eat in each meal and snack. It helps you create a calorie deficit, which is essential for losing body fat. By controlling portion sizes, you can regulate your calorie intake and ensure that you're not overeating. Here's how it works:

1. **Calorie Control**: Consuming fewer calories than your body needs for its daily functions leads to fat loss. Portion control helps you eat just the right amount of calories to create a deficit.

2. **Awareness**: Portion control encourages you to be more mindful of what you're eating. It can help you recognize when you're full and prevent overeating.

3. **Flexibility**: You can still enjoy a variety of foods in moderation, which makes it easier to stick to a long-term, sustainable eating plan.

4. **Avoiding Excess**: Large portions can lead to excess calorie intake, even if you're eating healthy foods. Controlling portions ensures you don't consume unnecessary calories.

5. **Regulation**: It helps regulate the balance between the number of calories you consume and the number of calories you burn through physical activity and metabolism.

6. **Smarter Choices**: Portion control encourages you to choose nutrient-dense foods that can keep you full and satisfied with smaller portions.

Incorporating portion control into your fat loss plan can be an effective and practical way to manage your weight and achieve your health goals. It's essential to combine it with a balanced diet, regular exercise, and other healthy lifestyle choices for optimal results.

FIFTH PRINCIPLE OF FAT LOSS:
Nutrient Quality

Opt for nutrient-dense foods, such as fruits, vegetables, lean proteins, and whole grains. These foods provide essential vitamins and minerals while helping you feel full with fewer calories.

Nutrient quality is a fundamental principle in fat loss because it focuses on the nutritional value of the foods you consume rather than just the number of calories. When you prioritize nutrient-dense foods, you can achieve fat loss more effectively for several reasons:

1. **Satiety**: Nutrient-dense foods, such as vegetables, lean proteins, and whole grains, are rich in fiber, vitamins, and minerals. These components promote a feeling of fullness and satisfaction, reducing the likelihood of overeating.

2. **Energy balance**: To lose fat, you need to maintain a calorie deficit (burn more calories than you consume). Nutrient-dense foods can help you achieve this by providing essential nutrients with fewer calories, making it easier to control your calorie intake.

3. **Metabolism**: Proper nutrition supports a healthy metabolism, which is essential for efficient fat loss. Nutrient-dense foods can help maintain and even boost your metabolic rate.

4. **Blood sugar control**: Foods with high nutrient quality, such as complex carbohydrates and lean proteins, can help stabilize blood sugar levels, reducing cravings and overeating.

5. **Muscle preservation**: During fat loss, you want to preserve lean muscle mass. Nutrient-dense foods provide the necessary protein and nutrients to support muscle maintenance.

6. **Nutrient balance**: A well-balanced diet ensures you get all the necessary vitamins and minerals, promoting overall health and well-being while losing fat.

In contrast, foods that are high in empty calories, such as sugary snacks and processed foods, can lead to excessive calorie intake and hinder your fat loss goals. Prioritizing nutrient quality in your diet can help you make sustainable, healthy choices that support fat loss while maintaining your overall health.

SIXTH PRINCIPLE OF FAT LOSS:
<u>Meal Timing</u>

The timing of meals and snacks can influence metabolism and hunger. Some people find success with strategies like intermittent fasting.

Meal timing is a principle of fat loss that focuses on when you consume your meals throughout the day. The idea behind it is to optimize your body's metabolism and energy expenditure to support fat loss. Here's how meal timing can influence fat loss:

- **Breakfast**: Eating a balanced breakfast can kickstart your metabolism and provide energy for the day. It helps prevent excessive hunger later, reducing the chances of overeating at other meals.

- **Frequent, Small Meals**: Some people advocate for eating smaller, more frequent meals throughout the day to maintain steady blood sugar levels and prevent excessive snacking or overeating.

- **Pre-Workout Nutrition**: Consuming a balanced meal or snack before a workout can provide energy, improve performance, and help you burn more calories during exercise.

- **Post-Workout Nutrition**: After a workout, your body can be more receptive to nutrients. Consuming a protein and carbohydrate-rich meal or shake can aid in recovery and muscle development, which indirectly supports fat loss.

- **Evening Eating**: Some experts recommend avoiding large meals close to bedtime as excess calories consumed late may not be utilized efficiently and could contribute to fat storage.

- **Caloric Distribution**: Regardless of the timing, it's essential to maintain a caloric deficit to lose fat. You need to burn more calories than you consume, and meal timing is just one aspect of achieving this deficit.

It's important to note that while meal timing can play a role in fat loss, it's not a magic solution on its own. The overall quality of your diet, portion sizes, and physical activity also significantly influence your ability to lose fat. Individual preferences and lifestyle should guide your meal timing choices, as what works best can vary from person to person.

SEVENTH PRINCIPLE OF FAT LOSS:
<u>Hydration</u>

Staying well-hydrated is important for overall health and can help control appetite.

Hydration is an important principle of fat loss because it plays a significant role in several aspects of the body's metabolism and overall health. Here's how hydration is related to fat loss:

- **Appetite control**: Dehydration can sometimes be mistaken for hunger, leading to overeating or snacking when you're actually thirsty. Staying well-hydrated can help you differentiate between thirst and true hunger, which can prevent unnecessary calorie consumption.

- **Metabolism**: Proper hydration is essential for efficient metabolism. When you're dehydrated, your body's metabolic rate may slow down, making it more challenging to burn calories and fat. Adequate hydration helps your metabolism function optimally.

- **Fat breakdown**: Water is necessary for the breakdown of fat molecules in the body. Dehydration can impair this process, making it harder to release stored fat for energy. Drinking enough water supports the body's ability to use fat as a fuel source.

- **Exercise performance**: Staying hydrated is crucial for maintaining physical performance during workouts. When you're dehydrated, you may feel fatigued and have reduced endurance, which can hinder your ability to engage in effective fat-burning exercise.

- **Thermoregulation**: Proper hydration helps regulate body temperature, especially during exercise. When your body overheats due to dehydration, it can negatively impact your exercise intensity and the effectiveness of your fat loss routine.

- **Detoxification**: Hydration is essential for the kidneys and liver to effectively remove waste and toxins from the body. When you're well-hydrated, these organs can function optimally, which is important for overall health and fat loss.

To support fat loss, it's generally recommended to drink an adequate amount of water throughout the day. The specific amount varies from person to person but aiming for around 8-10 cups (64-80 ounces) of water daily is a good starting point. It's important to note that hydration is just one aspect of a comprehensive fat loss plan, which should also include a balanced diet and regular physical activity.

EIGHTH PRINCIPLE OF FAT LOSS:
<u>Sleep and Stress Management</u>

Poor sleep and high stress levels can disrupt hormones related to hunger and satiety, making fat loss more challenging.

Sleep and rest management plays a crucial role in fat loss as it impacts various physiological and psychological aspects of weight management. Here's how it relates to fat loss as a principle:

- **Hormone Regulation**: Sleep is essential for maintaining hormonal balance. Lack of sleep can disrupt hormones like leptin (which controls hunger) and ghrelin (which stimulates appetite), leading to increased cravings and overeating, ultimately contributing to weight gain.

- **Metabolism**: Quality sleep promotes efficient metabolism. Sleep deprivation can slow down your metabolic rate, making it harder for your body to burn calories and fat.

- **Energy Levels**: Adequate rest ensures you have the energy and motivation to engage in physical activities, such as exercise. Regular exercise is crucial for fat loss, and lack of energy due to poor sleep can hinder your workout routine.

- **Stress Management**: Sleep and rest are essential for managing stress. High stress levels trigger the release of cortisol, a hormone that can lead to fat storage, especially around the abdominal area. Proper rest can help reduce stress and cortisol levels.

- **Recovery**: Rest and sleep are vital for muscle recovery. Adequate rest allows your muscles to repair and grow after exercise, which, in turn, boosts your metabolism and helps in fat loss.

- **Mindful Eating**: Sleep-deprived individuals often make poor food choices and eat impulsively. Being well-rested can enhance your ability to make mindful and healthy food choices, which is essential for fat loss.

- **Long-term Commitment**: Consistent sleep patterns and rest management contribute to overall well-being and create a sustainable foundation for fat loss. Sleep deprivation can lead to fatigue and increase the likelihood of giving in to unhealthy cravings and setbacks in your weight loss journey.

In summary, proper sleep and rest management are essential principles for fat loss because they regulate hormones, support metabolism, provide energy for exercise, reduce stress, aid in muscle recovery, and promote mindful eating. Incorporating healthy sleep habits into your weight loss plan is crucial for achieving and maintaining your desired fat loss goals.

NINTH PRINCIPLE OF FAT LOSS:
Exercise

A combination of cardio and strength training is effective for fat loss. Cardio burns calories, while strength training helps build muscle, which can boost metabolism.

Exercise is a key principle in the context of fat loss because it can help create a calorie deficit, which is essential for shedding body fat. Here's how it works:

- **Calorie expenditure**: When you engage in physical activity, your body burns calories for energy. This includes both structured workouts and everyday activities like walking, cleaning, and standing.

- **Muscle maintenance**: Exercise, especially resistance training, helps preserve and build lean muscle mass. More muscle means a higher resting metabolic rate, so you burn more calories even at rest.

- **Cardiovascular exercise**: Activities like running, swimming, or cycling can elevate your heart rate, increasing calorie burn during the exercise and potentially leading to afterburn effects (burning extra calories post-workout).

- **Appetite regulation**: Some people find that exercise can help control appetite and reduce cravings, making it easier to maintain a calorie deficit through dietary choices.

However, it's important to note that while exercise is beneficial, it's not a silver bullet for fat loss. Nutrition also plays a significant role. To lose fat effectively, it's essential to combine exercise with a balanced diet that creates a sustainable calorie deficit. Additionally, individual factors like genetics, metabolism, and hormones can influence the rate and effectiveness of fat loss through exercise.

TENTH PRINCIPLE OF FAT LOSS:
Individual Variation

Everyone's body responds differently to diet and exercise. What works for one person may not work for another, so it's important to find an approach that suits your needs and preferences.

Individual variation in the context of fat loss refers to the fact that different people may experience different rates of progress and outcomes when attempting to lose body fat. This principle recognizes that there are various factors that can influence how a person's body responds to fat loss efforts, including genetics, metabolism, lifestyle, and overall health. Some key points to consider regarding individual variation in fat loss:

- **Genetics**: Genetic factors play a significant role in determining a person's predisposition to gain or lose fat. Some individuals may have a genetic advantage when it comes to fat loss, while others may struggle more due to genetic factors.

- **Metabolism**: Metabolic rate can vary between individuals, and a faster metabolism can make it easier to burn calories and lose fat more quickly.

- **Lifestyle**: A person's daily habits, such as diet and physical activity, can greatly impact the rate of fat loss. People with similar genetics and metabolism can still experience different results based on their lifestyle choices.

- **Hormonal Factors**: Hormones play a crucial role in fat regulation. Variations in hormone levels, such as insulin and cortisol, can affect how the body stores and burns fat.

- **Adherence**: The ability to stick to a fat loss plan can vary among individuals. Some people may find it easier to adhere to a diet and exercise regimen, while others may struggle with consistency.

- **Stress and Sleep**: Stress levels and quality of sleep can impact fat loss. High stress and poor sleep quality may hinder progress for some individuals.

- **Age and Gender**: Age and gender can also influence fat loss. Men and younger individuals may have an advantage in terms of fat loss compared to women and older individuals due to differences in muscle mass and hormones.

Understanding and accommodating for individual variation is essential when designing a fat loss program. What works well for one person may not be equally effective for another, and a personalized approach that considers these factors is often the most successful in achieving sustainable fat loss.

ELEVENTH PRINCIPLE OF FAT LOSS:
Monitoring Progress

Tracking your food intake, physical activity, and progress can help you stay on track and make necessary adjustments.

Monitoring progress is a fundamental principle of fat loss because it helps individuals track their journey, stay motivated, and make necessary adjustments to their approach. Here's how it works:

- **Goal Setting**: To effectively lose fat, you need to set specific, measurable, and achievable goals. These could be related to body weight, body fat percentage, or clothing size.

- **Regular Assessment**: Regularly measure and assess your progress. This can include weighing yourself, taking body measurements, and tracking changes in your appearance and how your clothes fit.

- **Food and Activity Journal**: Keep a record of your food intake and physical activity. This can help you identify patterns, make better food choices, and optimize your workouts.

- **Monitoring Caloric Intake**: Be aware of your daily calorie consumption and macronutrient balance. Tracking what you eat can highlight areas where you may need to make adjustments to create a caloric deficit for fat loss.

- **Fitness Progress**: Keep track of your fitness achievements, such as increased strength, endurance, or improved workout performance. These are positive indicators of progress.

- **Consistency**: Consistency is key. Regular monitoring helps you stay accountable to your goals and maintain a consistent effort over time.

- **Adjustments**: If you're not making the expected progress, monitoring allows you to make informed adjustments. This might involve modifying your diet, exercise routine, or lifestyle factors.

- **Motivation**: Seeing positive changes and reaching milestones can boost motivation and reinforce your commitment to fat loss.

- **Mental Health**: Monitoring progress also extends to your mental well-being. Pay attention to how you feel mentally and emotionally, as fat loss can sometimes be a challenging journey.

- **Support System**: Share your progress with a supportive community or a fitness coach, as they can provide guidance and motivation.

Overall, monitoring progress is a powerful tool in the fat loss process, helping you stay on track, adapt to changing circumstances, and ultimately reach your goals more effectively.

Chapter 9

THE INNER AND OUTER GAMES OF HEALTH AND FITNESS

A training program lasting three months has a certain supernatural quality. That's when a lot of folks give up. Yes, oddly enough, throughout the years, I've witnessed scores of folks make it to three or four months before abruptly disappearing for various reasons. A few fell ill and never came back. Some chose to take a week off and make it an ongoing vacation. Some stopped caring about staying in shape because they were just lazy and began coming up with reasons.

One factor connected the majority of these individuals: they weren't satisfied with their accomplishments, and it makes sense that their drive declined in the absence of evidence of their labors. Fortunately, this is not going to be an issue for you. After three months, if you adhere to every tip in this book, you'll have made amazing progress and will be much more driven than you are now.

I want you to know that there are two equally vital components to getting the physique of your dreams before we get into the specifics of nutrition and training. I call these aspects the "outer game" and "inner game" of training.

The physical aspects of lifting, eating, sleeping, and other activities comprise the outer game, which is the main focus of most trainers, books, and periodicals. The less talked about part of training is the inner game, and if you don't have this under control, you're going to have a difficult time.

Naturally, the mental component of nutrition and exercise is the inner game, and it is this that truly distinguishes excellent physiques from mediocre ones. Developing a killer physique requires a disciplined, ordered approach to body maintenance, which is a significant lifestyle shift for most people. It does not involve following the latest fitness craze for a few months.

The inner and outer games of health and fitness refer to the psychological and physical aspects of maintaining a healthy lifestyle.

Inner Game:
- **Psychological factors**: This includes motivation, mindset, and self-discipline. The inner game involves setting goals, staying committed, and overcoming mental barriers that can hinder your progress.
- **Emotions and beliefs**: Understanding your emotions and addressing any limiting beliefs about your health and fitness can play a significant role in achieving your goals.
- **Self-awareness**: Being in tune with your body's needs and limitations is essential. This involves recognizing when to rest, when to push yourself, and when to seek help or guidance.

Outer Game:
- **Physical aspects**: This includes exercise, nutrition, and rest. Regular physical activity and a balanced diet are crucial for achieving and maintaining good health and fitness.
- **Environment**: Your surroundings, access to fitness facilities, and the people you surround yourself with can influence your health and fitness journey.
- **Techniques and strategies**: Utilizing proper workout techniques, following nutritional guidelines, and employing effective training strategies are key components of the outer game.

Note: Balancing the inner and outer games is essential for long-term success in health and fitness. A strong inner game can help you stay motivated and disciplined, while the outer game involves the practical steps you take to achieve your health and fitness goals.

Chapter 10

HOW TO SET FITNESS OBJECTIVES THAT WILL INSPIRE YOU

This seems so obvious and overdone, but it needs to be said nonetheless: You need to have clear, measurable objectives in mind before you lift weights, use a treadmill, or burn calories.

Individuals who have undefined, impractical, or uninspired exercise or health objectives—or none at all—quit first. They are also rather visible. They appear out of the blue and appear to sleepwalk through their training exercises, moving from machine to machine and simply performing the motions. They gripe about their inability to lose weight and lament how difficult it is to follow a diet week after week.

I can promise you that everyone with the kind of body you want has very clear, attainable goals for their fitness and health, and they are motivated by these goals to make small but steady progress toward them every day. To stay motivated, they set new goals after achieving the previous ones. In this chapter, I'm going to work this out for you.

Individuals rain for a variety of causes. Some people enjoy the challenge of challenging their bodies' boundaries. Some desire to appear well in order to win over the other sex. Some people desire greater self-confidence. Some people desire health and well-being.

In actuality, each of these arguments makes sense for training. The crucial thing is that you work out precisely what excites you about training. Sure, I could give you an endless list of advantages of being in fantastic shape, including looking great, feeling great, having high energy, being highly resistant to illness and disease, and so on.

We might as well begin with the element that most people value most highly: the visual. Hey, this isn't anything to be embarrassed about. I know of no one who has developed an incredible body without at least somewhat being driven by their desire to look a certain way.

Although pursuing appearances at all costs and disregarding one's health might lead to drug use and other bad habits, there is nothing wrong with being driven solely by the desire to look a specific way. I wouldn't be telling the truth if I said I didn't care as much about appearances, but I do respect my health and am not just motivated by vanity. Being slender and muscular makes me feel fantastic, and I love how I look in the mirror.

STEP 1:
WHAT KIND OF BODY DO YOU DREAM OF HAVING?

Choosing the type of body you aspire to have is the first step towards setting objectives. Not in your imagination, but in actuality. You must locate images of people with the physique type you like and store them for later use.

It may seem absurd for you to go online and look at images of individuals, but it's crucial that you have a precise mental picture of the type of body you want. Seeing images of actual bodies that you aspire to own can and will help you stay motivated.

STEP 2:
WHAT IS THE PERFECT HEALTH STATE IN YOUR OPINION?

After determining your ideal appearance, let's examine the second aspect of this equation: health. If your main reason for training is to look a specific way, you will quickly discover that the health advantages are just as compelling. Better physical and mental health, increased vitality, increased strength, increased sex desire, and increased mental alertness are all expected benefits.

Determine a health objective that inspires you. My goal is similar to this: to have a long-lasting, robust, disease-free, and lively body that enables me to be active and fully enjoy life. That seems to be the main focus of this for me. I want to be well, live a long life, see my future children grow up, and never experience a crippling illness.

Your interests in health are undoubtedly similar to mine, but you are free to formulate your own objectives in any language that speaks most to you.

<u>STEP 3:</u>
WHY DO YOU WANT TO ACHIEVE THESE GOALS?

Okay, so you've determined your desired appearance and degree of health. The next question is, "Why?" Why have those objectives been accomplished? Write whatever inspires you the most; this is entirely personal.

Perhaps you want to feel more confident; perhaps you want to improve at the physically demanding hobbies or sports you play; perhaps you want to attract more attention from the other sex; perhaps you want to be able to engage in physical activities with your children; perhaps you just want to be able to perform a few pull-ups. Whatever your motivations, simply make a list of them all.

Write the "whys" for the appearances first for the purpose of simplicity, and then concentrate on the health objective.

THE FINAL WORD

These three easy procedures will have given you a strong "motivation sheet" that will guide you at all times. You can glance at that sheet and likely alter your mind while you're reading the gym and feeling a little fatigued. You'll understand exactly why you're eating your fish and veggies when you're out with buddies and you see them gorge themselves.

Some Bodybuilders have been using this straightforward yet effective approach to sustain their motivation to exercise and follow a diet. Their objectives have evolved over the years, they always made sure they knew where there were heading and why. It's likely that you will gain a great deal from young as well.

Chapter 11

TRAINING WITH A GOOD PARTNER

Working out with a dedicated partner can be a highly motivating and rewarding experience. Whether you're an experienced lifter or just starting your fitness journey, having a reliable workout partner can bring numerous benefits. Together, you can push each other to new limits, spot each other during challenging lifts, and provide the necessary encouragement to stay consistent in your training. This camaraderie not only enhances your physical progress but also makes the entire fitness journey more enjoyable. In this conversation, we'll explore the advantages and tips for successful bodybuilding partnerships.

Working out with a good partner in bodybuilding can be beneficial in several ways:

1. **Motivation**: A workout partner can provide motivation and encouragement, pushing you to give your best during each session.

2. **Spotting**: Having a partner can be essential for safety during heavy lifts, as they can spot you and help prevent injury.

3. **Accountability**: Knowing that someone is relying on you to show up at the gym can help you stay consistent with your training.

4. **Variety**: Partner workouts can introduce new exercises and training techniques, adding variety to your routine.

5. **Friendly competition**: A bit of healthy competition with your partner can drive both of you to achieve better results.

However, it's essential to choose a partner who has similar goals and dedication to avoid potential conflicts or distractions during your workouts. Communication and coordination are key for a successful training partnership.

Working out with a bad workout partner in bodybuilding can be frustrating and counterproductive. A bad partner may lack motivation, be unreliable, or not provide the support and encouragement you need. It's essential to communicate openly with your partner and consider whether it's better to train alone or find a more compatible training partner to help you achieve your fitness goals effectively.

Working out with a bad partner in bodybuilding can have several negative consequences:

1. **Poor form and technique**: A bad workout partner may not provide proper guidance or feedback on your form and technique, which can lead to incorrect movements and increase the risk of injury.

2. **Inconsistent motivation**: If your partner lacks commitment or motivation, it can be demotivating for you and hinder your progress. Consistency is crucial in bodybuilding.

3. **Wasted time**: Inefficient workouts due to a bad partner can lead to wasted time and effort in the gym, as you may not be targeting the right muscle groups or achieving your goals effectively.

4. **Plateauing**: A subpar workout partner may not push you to reach your full potential, which can result in hitting a plateau and not making the desired gains.

5. **Safety concerns**: If your partner doesn't prioritize safety and proper spotting, there's an increased risk of accidents and injuries during heavy lifts.

6. **Conflicting goals**: Misalignment in goals and training preferences can lead to conflicts and hinder your ability to follow a consistent training program.

It's essential to communicate with your workout partner and ensure that you both have similar goals, commitment levels, and a focus on safety and proper form to maximize the benefits of your bodybuilding workouts.

Chapter 12

YOU CANNOT KNOW ANYTHING IF YOU CANNOT MEASURE IT

"You Cannot Know Anything If You Cannot Measure It" is a fundamental concept in the world of bodybuilding workouts. This principle emphasizes the importance of quantifying and tracking various aspects of your training and progress to achieve optimal results. By measuring factors such as weight lifted, repetitions, body measurements, and nutrition intake, bodybuilders can make informed decisions, set realistic goals, and fine-tune their workout routines to maximize muscle growth, strength gains, and overall fitness. This approach highlights the significance of data-driven training and self-assessment in the pursuit of a well-defined and sculpted physique.

A brilliant scientist and engineer by the name of Sir William Thomson, sometimes referred to as Lord Kelvin, once stated that knowledge is incomplete if one cannot quantify or articulate numbers about a subject.

It turns out that training and dieting can benefit greatly from this information. You can determine if you're moving in the correct path or not if you can quantify our progress—or lack thereof—and communicate actual numbers. You're winging it and crossing your fingers if you don't have a mechanism to gauge progress.

Maintaining a training and nutrition journal is among the best defenses against becoming stuck and making no progress. This might seem excessive at first, but believe me—it makes a big difference. It is, in my opinion, Italy's long-term gain.

Allow me to pose a query to you. What aspects of their training and dieting are they finding the most frustrating? Getting caught in a rut and reaching a plateau is, without a doubt, the answer to that question. There is nothing more inconvenient than dedicating the same amount of time and energy to working out every day, week after week.

What about diets, then? What is it about this place that frustrates you the most? not gaining muscle or dropping weight as rapidly as they need to. Many people believe they are eating healthily, yet they aren't developing much muscle or losing much fat for "inexplicable" reasons.

It's nearly a given that you will have these issues if you don't maintain a training and nutrition log. You will hit a training plateau and always struggle to eat healthfully, especially when it comes to weight loss. How come?

THE TRAINING JOURNAL

Gaining the body of your dreams takes time. It's a marathon, not a sprint, as they say. Regardless of how you look at it, it requires a significant time and effort investment. However, if you know what you're doing, you can earn amazing results and enjoy the trip.

Getting stronger is the secret to building muscle. Your muscles need to grow in order to get stronger and able to handle ever greater weights. The tough thing about muscle strength now is that it develops gradually. When you first start out, your strength will increase dramatically over the course of the first few months, but then it will start to taper down. You will have to actively work for each pound of progress on your lifts after that. This is, of course, where things become murky for those who don't maintain diaries, and they eventually find themselves stuck in a weekly cycle of doing the same workouts with the same weights and repetitions. This is a terrific technique to not make any progress at all, along with the fact that you can't assess any improvement at all and you have to perform various exercises with random weights every week.

How can one prevent this? That's the purpose of your journal. Every week, try to do a little bit more than you did the week before. This does not necessarily translate into gaining more weight because it would be impractical to increase weight for every exercise every week. Reps are also included. Eventually, more reps translate into more weight. For instance, you should be able to come in on week four and perform 8 reps of 100–105 pounds if you squatted 90 pounds for 8 reps on week one, 9 reps on week two, and 10 reps on week three. After then, the procedure is repeated up to 110 pounds, 115 pounds, and so forth. One rep at a time, this is the way strength is developed.

However, you most likely won't remember what you did the previous week if you don't keep a journal. Yes, you may mentally record the specific workouts, but what about the rest? Every exercise must be approached in the same manner. "One more rep!" should be your motto. Give yourself a pat on the back if you can complete an exercise with one more rep than you did the previous week (with appropriate form). You've come a long way. Don't give up if you can't perform any better than the previous week; nonetheless, you must exert greater effort the following week. If you find yourself stuck for a few weeks, there's a problem and you should review your rest and nutrition.

HOW TO KEEP A TRAINING JOURNAL

How then do you maintain a training log? Extremely Easy. Alternatively, you may go old school and grab a notepad. I like to use Gym Buddy or JEFit, two applications you can get on your phone or iPod.

Write a list of the following in your notebook for each training day: the day, date, and body part(s) you will be training, as well as the number of weeks since your last rest week. Additionally, you should weigh yourself once or twice a week—in the morning, after using the restroom, on an empty stomach, and in the nude—and enter the results in your book.

Next, you make a list of the exercises from the previous week that you will review. You determine whether you're increasing the weight or the reps this week (you'll find out more about that shortly) and begin your first exercise, recording your form as you go. In this manner, you progress through your workout, constantly checking to make sure you are aiming to perform more repetitions or heavier weight than the previous week. Here's an example of how a training journal looks like:

Week 1
192 Ibs
8/14/11

Monday
Chest
Bench Press- 275 x 4, x 4, x 4 (feel stronger)
Incline Dumbbell Press - 110 x 5, x 5, x 4
Decline Dumbbell Press - 110 x 5, x 5, x 5

Pretty easy, huh? Make notes sometimes if you are feeling very strong or weak during an activity, if a set was difficult for you, if you have an ache or pain, if you had a difficult night's sleep, etc.

Maintaining your notebook in this manner enables you to stay focused on progress at all times, avoid regressing or being stuck (and in the event that you do stumble, you can identify the precise causes and find solutions to assist you get out of a rut).

The training journal is essentially empty. Good apps give you nice graphs to display your progress along with the ability to track all the same things.

THE DIET JOURNAL

Keeping a bodybuilding diet journal can be a valuable tool to track your progress and stay on top of your nutrition. In your journal, consider including:

1. Daily Food Intake: Document everything you eat and drink throughout the day, including portion sizes.

2. Macronutrient Breakdown: Keep track of your protein, carbohydrates, and fat intake. This helps ensure you're meeting your nutritional goals.

3. Caloric Intake: Monitor your daily calorie consumption to maintain, gain, or lose weight based on your fitness goals.

4. Meal Timing: Note the timing of your meals and snacks. Some people benefit from specific meal timing strategies.

5. Hydration: Record your daily water intake. Staying hydrated is crucial for overall health and muscle function.

6. Supplements: If you take supplements, jot down the types and amounts. This includes protein powders, vitamins, or any other relevant supplements.

7. Workout Details: Include details about your workouts – exercises, sets, and reps. This can help you correlate nutrition with exercise performance.

8. How You Feel: Note your energy levels, mood, and any physical or mental changes. This can provide insights into the effects of your diet on your well-being.

9. Sleep Patterns: Your sleep can impact muscle recovery and overall health. Track your sleep duration and quality.

10. Reflections: Take a moment each day to reflect on your progress, challenges, and any adjustments you might want to make.

Consistency is key when maintaining a diet journal. It can help identify patterns, track successes, and pinpoint areas for improvement in your bodybuilding journey.

Now, for the actual journal itself, there are many phone, tablet, and web apps out there built for this, but I like to just use Word (or you can use Google's free version, found in their Google Drive app—love this app!). Many people have also used plain old notebooks.
Every day, jot down the following in your journal:

1. Your calorie, protein, carb, and fat intake goals.

2. The items you intend to eat, along with a breakdown of the calories, protein, carbohydrates, and fats in each meal.

3. A comment on whether or not you ate the scheduled meal. If you followed your plan, you may just mark the meal with a check mark; but, if you had to stray from it—which is something you should try to avoid, but occasionally it's unavoidable—you should record what you ate and include the calories, protein, carbohydrates, and fats.

This could appear like this:

15/11/2023
Monday

<u>Targets</u>
1,600 calories
150 grams of carbs
30 grams of fat
180 grams of protein

<u>Meals</u>
7:00AM Meal 1
(Pre workout meal)

1 cup of rice milk
30 grams of protein
30 grams of whey protein
25 grams of carbs
270 calories
6 grams of fat

9:00AM Meal 2
(Post workout smoothie)
1 cup of rice milk
2 bananas
30 grams of protein
1 scoop of protein powder
2.5 grams of fat
50 grams of carbs
342 calories

(And so forth, decomposing every meal, throughout the day.)

According to an old saying, "If you fail to plan, you plan to fail." This holds true for diet as well. Without planning and preparation in the manner I've just outlined, becoming thin and strong is practically impossible, which is why the majority of individuals don't get the desired outcomes.

Chapter 13

INTENSITY AND FOCUS: YOUR TWO SECRET WEAPONS

Intensity and focus are the dynamic duo that can elevate your performance and productivity to new heights. Intensity channels your energy, infusing tasks with vigor, while focus sharpens your mental acuity, enabling you to delve deep into the heart of challenges. Together, they form your secret weapons, empowering you to tackle goals with precision and purpose. Intensity and focus are indeed crucial in bodybuilding workouts. Intensity ensures you're pushing your limits, while focus ensures proper form and mind-muscle connection for optimal results. Combine them, and you have a powerful formula for effective training. Let's explore how cultivating these traits can unlock your full potential.

Intensity and focus are crucial in bodybuilding workouts for optimal results.

Intensity:
Definition: Intensity refers to the level of effort and exertion you put into your exercises during a workout.

Importance: High intensity stimulates muscle growth by causing micro-tears in muscle fibers, prompting the body to repair and strengthen them. This is essential for hypertrophy, or muscle size increase.

Application: Increase intensity by lifting heavier weights, reducing rest times between sets, and incorporating techniques like drop sets or supersets.

Focus:
Definition: Focus involves mental concentration on the muscle being worked and the exercise being performed.

Importance: A focused mindset enhances mind-muscle connection, ensuring that you activate and engage the target muscle effectively. This can lead to more controlled movements and better muscle recruitment.

Application: Concentrate on the quality of each repetition, visualize the muscle contracting, and minimize distractions to optimize the effectiveness of your workout.

Combining intensity and focus maximizes the efficiency of your bodybuilding routine, fostering muscle development and overall strength. Integrating these two elements helps create a purposeful and results-driven training experience.

Chapter 14

THE COMPONENTS OF A BALANCED DIET (NUTRITION)

A balanced diet consists of essential components that provide the necessary nutrients for overall health. These components include carbohydrates for energy, proteins for tissue repair, fats for energy storage, vitamins for various bodily functions, minerals for structural support, and water for hydration. Achieving a balance ensures proper growth, development, and maintenance of the body, supporting optimal functioning of organs and systems.

Here are the key components and their explanations:

CARBOHYDRATES

Carbohydrates are macronutrients that serve as a primary source of energy for the body. They include sugars, starches, and fibers, found in foods like fruits, grains, and vegetables.

Function: Primary energy source for the body.

Sources: Grains, fruits, vegetables, legumes.

CALORIES

Calories are a measure of the energy content in food. Consuming more calories than your body uses can lead to weight gain, while a calorie deficit may result in weight loss. It's essential to balance calorie intake with physical activity for overall health.

Function: Basic functions like breathing and circulation, as well as physical activities.

Sources: Calories come from three main macronutrients: carbohydrates (4 calories per gram), proteins (4 calories per gram), and fats (9 calories per gram). Alcohol also contributes calories (7 calories per gram), but it's not a nutrient essential for survival. Keep in mind that vitamins and minerals don't provide significant calories.

PROTEINS

Proteins are essential macromolecules composed of amino acids, playing crucial roles in cell structure, function, and regulation. They serve various functions, including enzymes for biochemical reactions, structural components, and signaling molecules in the body.

Function: Essential for tissue repair, enzyme production, and immune function.

Sources: Meat, poultry, fish, dairy, legumes, nuts.

FATS

Fats are essential macronutrients that play a crucial role in the body, serving as a source of energy, supporting cell structure, and aiding in the absorption of fat-soluble vitamins. There are different types of fats, including saturated fats, unsaturated fats, and trans fats, each with varying effects on health. It's important to maintain a balanced and healthy fat intake as part of a well-rounded diet.

Function: Provides energy, supports cell structure, and aids in the absorption of fat-soluble vitamins.

Sources: Avocado, nuts, seeds, olive oil, fatty fish.

VITAMINS

Vitamins are essential organic compounds that play crucial roles in various physiological functions within the body, promoting overall health and well-being. They are necessary for processes such as metabolism, immune function, and cellular repair. Vitamins are typically obtained through diet, as the body is unable to produce an adequate amount of them on its own.

Function: Essential for various metabolic processes and overall well-being.

Sources: Fruits, vegetables, dairy, meat, whole grains.

MINERALS

Minerals are essential micronutrients required by the human body for various physiological functions. They include elements such as calcium, iron, magnesium, zinc, and others. These minerals play crucial roles in bone health, nerve function, oxygen transport, and overall metabolic processes. Obtaining a balanced intake of minerals through a diverse diet is important for maintaining good health.

Function: Necessary for bone health, fluid balance, and nerve function.

Sources: Leafy greens, dairy, nuts, seeds, whole grains.

WATER

Water is a crucial component of food, providing hydration and contributing to various culinary processes. It influences the texture, juiciness, and overall sensory experience of foods.

Function: Vital for hydration, digestion, and nutrient transportation.

Sources: Beverages, fruits, vegetables.

FIBER

Fiber is a type of carbohydrate found in plant-based foods like fruits, vegetables, and whole grains. It's essential for digestive health, helps prevent constipation, and may contribute to lower cholesterol levels.

Function: Aids in digestion, helps prevent constipation, and may reduce the risk of certain diseases.

Sources: Whole grains, fruits, vegetables, legumes.

ANTIOXIDANTS

Antioxidants are compounds that help neutralize harmful molecules called free radicals in the body, potentially reducing oxidative stress and preventing damage to cells. Common sources include fruits, vegetables, and certain nuts.

Function: Protects cells from damage caused by free radicals, potentially reducing the risk of chronic diseases.

Sources: Berries, dark chocolate, spinach, nuts.

CALCIUM

Calcium is an essential mineral for building and maintaining strong bones and teeth. It also plays a crucial role in nerve transmission, muscle function, and blood clotting. Good dietary sources of calcium include dairy products, leafy green vegetables, and fortified foods.

Function: Essential for bone and teeth health, blood clotting, and muscle function.

Sources: Dairy products, leafy greens, fortified foods.

IRON

Iron is a crucial dietary mineral found in various foods. It plays a vital role in transporting oxygen through the blood and is an essential component of hemoglobin, the protein in red blood cells. Good food sources of iron include red meat, poultry, fish, beans, lentils, and fortified cereals.

Function: Critical for the formation of hemoglobin and oxygen transport in the blood.

Sources: Red meat, poultry, fish, beans, fortified cereals.

Remember, a balanced diet involves consuming these components in appropriate proportions to meet individual nutritional needs. It's also important to consider factors such as age, sex, physical activity, and any specific health conditions.

Chapter 15

EAT THIS, NOT THAT: BECOMING THINNER LEANER STRONGER VERSIONS

Eat This, Not That is the book, have you seen it? Choose the 540-calorie Big Mac over the 750-calorie Angus Deluxe and you will lose weight! Get skinny by consuming a Cold Stone Creamery Oreo Crème Ice Cream Sandwich rather than a Sinless Cake'n Shake Milkshake! Eat until you're slim! Get significant weight loss without ever hitting the gym!

I have to give the author credit for the concept, even though the book's explosive climb to fame is a sad testament to people's lack of willpower and misunderstanding of the body's true functions. For those who would rather make their own Banana-Rum Split than indulge in the 1,000-calorie Baskin Robbins version, this product was ideal for those looking to lose weight.

I'm going to give you Eat This, Not That in the Becoming Thinner, Leaner, Stronger form. We'll examine various forms of lipids, carbohydrates, and proteins, as well as which foods to eat and which to avoid, along with a few other dietary guidelines that will support you in reaching your fitness objectives.

SOURCES OF PROTEIN

Whole food protein and supplemented protein are the two primary forms or sources of protein available.

You guessed it: whole food protein is derived from real food sources like beef, poultry, fish, etc. Eggs, milk, fish, poultry, lean red meat, and turkey are the finest sources of whole food protein. The finest foods for vegetarians are eggs, low-fat Greek yogurt (0%Fage is my favorite brand), low-fat cottage cheese (Organic Valley is my favorite brand), tempeh, tofu, quinoa, almonds, rice, and beans.

While we're talking about vegetarianism, some people assert that in order to guarantee that your body is receiving "complete" proteins—that is, proteins that have all of the amino acids required to form tissue—you must properly combine your proteins whether you're a vegetarian or vegan. The Massachusetts Institute of Technology comprehensively disproved this idea and the flawed research it was founded on, but it persists. Although it is true that some vegetable protein sources contain less of a given amino acid than other protein sources, there isn't any scientific proof to support the claim that they are completely devoid of them.

The three most frequent sources of protein supplements are eggs, soy, and whey—a liquid left over after milk is squeezed and curdled during the cheese-making process. Protein supplements can also be powdered or liquid foods. Additionally, there are excellent plant-based supplements available that combine high-quality protein sources including hemp, peas, quinoa, brown rice, and fruit.

Although obtaining all of your protein from whole foods may not be feasible for certain people, protein powder is a simple alternative. You don't need any supplements to eat healthily.

There are a few things you should be aware of regarding protein consumption presently. The first topic is the amount of protein that can be absorbed in a single session. Studies on this subject are highly controversial and conflicting, primarily due to the complexity of the topic. A person's lean mass, lifestyle, metabolism, digestive tract health, and heredity are all significant contributors. To keep things simple, though, here's what I know: you can consume and utilize a lot of protein at each meal. To be accurate, how much? It should be easy for your body to absorb up to 60 grams in a single sitting.

Although there are no advantages to eating this manner (in fact, I find bingeing to be rather uncomfortable), it's helpful to know in case you skip a meal and have to make it up by adding a lot of protein to a subsequent meal.

It's also important to understand that different proteins digest at different rates and that the body uses some proteins more effectively than others. For example, the body uses 70–80% of the protein in beef, which is rapidly digested (the precise percentage varies depending on which study you read, but they all lie between 70% and 80%). Additionally, whey protein digests quickly. Depending on the study you read, its "net protein utilization," or how the body uses the protein, ranges from 90 to 95%. Compared to whey and beef, egg protein digests somewhat more slowly, yet its NPU is in the same range.

Understanding NPU and digestion speeds is crucial because you should consume high-NPU proteins to fulfill your daily protein needs. You should also plan to have a slow-digesting protein for your last meal before bed and a quick-digesting protein for your post-workout meal.

These options are yours:

<u>WHOLE FOOD PROTEINS</u>

Lean meats (pork, chicken, beef, and turkey)
Fish
Eggs
Vegetarian sources noted above

<u>PROTEINS SUPPLEMENTS</u>

Egg
Whey
Casein
High-quality plant-based protein supplements

If you're wondering why I didn't include soy protein in my list of suggested supplements, it's because of the debate around its impact on hormones. Studies have indicated that frequent soy eating may raise estrogen levels. I know that studies have shown the contrary to be true—that frequent soy eating has no feminizing effects on men—but I decided to wait for further data before making my decision. The fact that the majority of soy protein supplements come from genetically engineered soybeans bothers me as well.

Now, as for when to eat slow- or fast-digesting proteins, I suggest consuming whey, a fast-digesting protein, after a workout to boost blood levels of amino acids (and thus promote muscle growth), and egg or case, a slow-digesting protein, thirty minutes before bed, as this has been shown to enhance muscle recovery. You can have whey or egg for the remaining meals that you supplement with. Since too much whey makes me bloated, I like to take supplements made of eggs.

TYPES OF CARBOHYDRATES

Consuming enough carbohydrates each day is essential for building muscle and strength. In addition to providing energy for your workouts and allowing you to appropriately overload your muscles, carbohydrates are essential for pre- and post-workout meals.

Having said that, most carbohydrates consumed by the majority of people are not only harmful due to their high GI and genetically modified substances, but they are also highly processed.
The typical snack items are shown below along with their average GI scores. There is some, but not significant, variation in the GI scores across brands.

(The University of Sydney, the University of Harvard, and Livestrong.com are the sources of the information below.)

FOOD	GI
Corn chips	63
White bread bagel	72
Pretzels	83
Breakfast cereal like cornflakes, Raisin Bran, Special K etc.	72-84
Corn cracker or wheat	67-87
Candy bar	62-78
Popcorn	72
Rice cake	78
Rye crackers.	64
Cornflakes	93
Pizza	80
White rice	64
White bread	70
While wheat bread	71
English muffin (white bread)	77
Instant oatmeal	83
Baked potato	85
Coca cola	63
Baguette	95

I can understand if finding a lot of your favorite snacks on that list makes you feel a little sad. Sadly, if you want a lean, vital body and high, consistent energy levels, these foods just cannot be consumed frequently enough.

There's a straightforward guideline to stick to when it comes to high-, medium-, and low-glycemic carbohydrates, regardless of how many you need to consume daily (depending on what your body is trying to accomplish).

Eat carbs within thirty minutes of finishing your workout, but preferably in the medium-high range of the glycemic index (70–90 is a good starting point). (I'll figure out the precise quantities for you shortly.)

You require enough energy for your training, which is why you desire some carbohydrates before you work out. Your muscles are famished for glycogen, so you want to replenish it as soon as possible to keep your body in an anabolic state and prevent muscle atrophy.

Bananas and rice milk are my favorite pre- and post-workout carbohydrates, but unprocessed items on the above high-GI list, like baked potatoes, white rice, instant oatmeal, and fruits with glycemic index values above 60, like cantaloupe, pineapple, watermelon, dates, apricots, and figs, are also excellent options. Because table sugar (sucrose) has a high GI, some people advise eating it after working out, but I try to avoid processed sugar as much as possible.

Your other carbs should all fall into one of two categories on the glycemic index: low or moderate (60 and below is a decent rule of thumb). It really is that easy. Following this guideline can help you avoid a plethora of issues that other people experience as a result of the highs and lows in energy that occur with consuming high-GI carbohydrates on a regular basis, as well as disease.

Here are a few examples of delicious and healthful carbohydrates you may incorporate into your diet:

FOOD	GI
Multi-grain muffin	45
Multi-grain braed	43
Whole grain sourdough bread	48
Brown rice	55
Basmati rice	43
Yam	37
Apple	36
Peanuts	14
Black beans	30
Almonds	10
Orange	43

Blackberries	32
Strawberries	40
Oatmeal	58

Therefore, throw out items such as sugar, white bread, processed, low-quality whole wheat bread, junk food, crackers, waffls, and cornflakes, as well as junk cereas and muffins. For your body's sake, I would even advise against consuming these processed food kinds as pre- or post-workout carbohydrates.

Even some fruits, including dates and watermelon, are poor choices for daily snacks due to their high glycemic index ratings. If you're not sure where a carb you enjoy fits on the glycemic index, do some research on it. Simply avoid including it in any meals that aren't right before or right after doing exercise if it's more than 60.

TYPES OF FATS

To ensure you get enough fat per day, focus on incorporating healthy fats into your diet. Include sources like avocados, nuts, seeds, olive oil, and fatty fish. Aim for a balanced intake, considering both saturated and unsaturated fats, while staying within your daily caloric needs. Consulting with a nutritionist can provide personalized guidance based on your individual requirements and health goals.

Getting enough healthy fats everyday is very easy and simple. The rules goes like this;

- Understand your daily caloric requirements and ensure that an appropriate percentage comes from healthy fats.

- Incorporate a diverse range of fats, such as monounsaturated fats (e.g., olive oil), polyunsaturated fats (e.g., fatty fish, seeds), and limited saturated fats.

- Be mindful of portion sizes to avoid excessive caloric intake, as fats are calorie-dense. Balance your fat intake with other essential nutrients.

- Prioritize sources of healthy fats, such as avocados, nuts, seeds, and fatty fish, while minimizing intake of trans fats and highly processed oils.

- Aim for a balanced diet that includes adequate amounts of carbohydrates, proteins, and fats, ensuring overall nutritional equilibrium.

Ensuring an adequate intake of healthy fats is crucial for overall well-being. Incorporating sources like avocados, nuts, and olive oil can support heart health, brain function, and nutrient absorption. However, moderation is key, as excessive fat intake may lead to weight-related issues. It's essential to strike a balance within daily caloric needs for optimal health.

Chapter 16

MEAL PLANNING TIPS TO HELP YOU ACHIEVE YOUR GOALS

Meal plans for many people are designed to make them gain weight. They skip breakfast, consume junk food at noon, return home ravenous, have a large dinner with dessert, and then spend the evening munching on popcorn or chips while watching TV. This is precisely how you add layers of unsightly fat and destroy your metabolism.

This chapter will cover the fundamentals of planning your daily food schedule.

MACRO-NUTRIENT PLANNING

<u>CARBOHYDRATES</u>

You should consume the majority of your daily carbs before and after exercise, as this is when your body need them most.

I also want to talk about the issue of consuming carbohydrates a few hours before bed. This advice has been around for a while in the fitness and health community, but usually with the incorrect justification.

Eating carbohydrates right before bed or at night does not seem to cause weight gain, but it may prevent fat loss. How?

The body quits using fat as an energy source by producing insulin to digest and absorb the carbohydrates that are consumed. Since your body burns fat at its highest rate while you sleep, it stands to reason that high insulin levels before bed could hinder fat loss.

This is related to the finding that research has shown that insulin synthesis and processing interfere with growth hormone synthesis, which has potent fat-burning properties. As your body naturally produces a large amount of growth hormone while you sleep, increased insulin levels before bed may also negatively impact your body's ability to manufacture growth hormone, depriving you of its fat-burning properties.

Although there isn't much research on this topic right now, I limit my carbohydrate intake after supper because I don't think it's necessary to consume a lot of them before bed when I'm cutting. When I go to bed, I want my insulin levels to be as close to baseline as feasible.

PROTEIN

Protein should be consumed every three to five hours. Studies have revealed that the body's anabolic reaction to protein consumption lasts approximately five hours, thus you should never go home for more than five hours without eating protein. This means you should consume enough protein at each meal to reach your nutritional goals and 4-6 times a day.

FATS

Your fat intake can be distributed throughout the day. I like to start my day with 1-2 tablespoons of Udo's oil, which is a fantastic 3-6-9 blend, but you are under no need to purchase it. All you have to do is stick to the good fat sources I mentioned before.

THE PRE-WORK MEAL:30-20-20

You should have 20 grams of high-GI carbohydrates and 20 grams of quickly digested protein, such as whey, around 30 minutes before to doing out.

In addition to providing you with energy to power your exercise, carbohydrates also cause the production of insulin, which blocks the effects of cortisol and, in a University of Oklahoma research, boosts protein synthesis and blood supply to the muscles.

When you begin to break down your muscle fibers by lifting weights, the protein will deliver amino acids into your bloodstream, where they can be used right away for repair.

THE POST-WORKOUT MEAL

A lot of people are shocked to hear how crucial it is to have a meal after working out.

Studies have indicated that consuming carbohydrates and protein following weight training promotes increased muscle growth and enhances exercise efficiency in subsequent sessions.

Your body will absorb glucose, glycogen, and amino acids more quickly than usual after workout. Should you eat within this "window," you will be squandering a chance to advance toward your objectives more quickly.

As a result, it's crucial to eat within an hour or two of concluding your weight exercise, and to have a healthy balance of carbohydrates and protein.

It's important to remember that the aforementioned suggestions should be followed following weight training, not before. As cardio does not drain glycogen stores like weight training does, you do not need to load up on carbohydrates after a cardio workout. The only exception is if you're doing prolonged, high-intensity cardio—one that involves more than an hour of sprinting or other anaerobic exercise. Nevertheless, in order to reduce muscle breakdown, I prefer to have some protein before doing cardio.

PRE-SLEEP MEAL

The final meal of the evening should be a slow-digesting protein, and it should be eaten right before bed. Studies have indicated that this maintains an increase in amino acids throughout the slumber, which can subsequently be utilized to sustain muscle healing during the night. It expedites the healing of your muscles.

For my pre-sleep protein, I like egg protein powder, low-fat cottage cheese, or Greek yogurt with no added fat. Casein is another popular option.

WHAT TO EAT DURING YOUR FREE DAYS

You don't need to worry about cutting calories on days when you don't train.Though it would seem reasonable since you expend less calories on those days, in actuality, it won't matter if you cut them back or not.

As I train early in the morning, the only adjustment I make on days off is to skip my elegant post-workout meal, which serves as breakfast. Rather, I typically consume the same number of calories and carbohydrates with protein sources like eggs, protein shakes, fat-free yogurt, and hot cereals like oatmeal.

Great eating habits are essential to building a great body. You already know what that entails: eating the correct amounts of calories, protein, carbs, and fats on the right schedule, as well as drinking enough water to make sure your body has everything it needs to adapt to the rigorous training you put it through.

Chapter 17

YOUR BECOME THINNER LEANER STRONGER DIET PLAN

Understanding how many calories to consume daily and what proportion of those calories should come from fats, carbohydrates, and proteins is essential for following a healthy diet.

That's what this chapter is all about, though: figuring out how to precisely calculate your food needs for both weight loss and "maintaining," or eating in a way that allows you to add muscle steadily but without gaining any fat.

Calorie and macro objectives can be calculated using a variety of formulas and techniques. Some are predicated on the notion that eating ought to happen where you want to be, not where you are right now. Although I've found these strategies to be effective, one potential drawback is that they require you to know your body fat %. Scales that "measure" body fat levels and handheld electrical devices that purport to calculate body fat percentages can both be incredibly incorrect. In nearly every situation, taking measurements and entering them into an online body fat percentage calculator will get wildly erroneous answers.

That being said, the diet calculation approach I'm about to offer with you is based on your present body weight and goal (either losing weight or gradually gaining muscle while gaining little to no fat). It's pretty doable and straightforward. If you're curious about your body fat %, the majority of experts concur that the most reliable ways to find out are through hydrostatic testing, DEXA x-rays, and Bod Pod testing. The drawbacks are expense and inconvenience, though.

That's why I advise you to purchase a high-quality fat caliper. Accurate measurements can be obtained by appropriately using this straightforward gadget during testing.

MAXIMUM FAT LOSS DIETING

Reducing your daily calorie intake is all that is necessary to lose fat, and as you will discover, cutting your carbs accounts for the majority of the calories you eliminate from your diet.

Maintaining your current weight is easier than losing it since you are trying to keep your caloric intake at a level that will allow you to shed fat steadily while losing as little muscle and strength as possible. You run the risk of losing muscle if you consume a little too little or too much each day, which will impede your efforts to lose weight.

If this is your first time trying to lose weight, I would like to caution you that the first couple of weeks can be challenging. You will experience hunger and a desire for carbohydrates. It simply is what it is. But if you persevere, the second week will go much more smoothly for you. You won't even notice by week four or five.

Figuring Out Your Diet For Weight Loss

Your diet will be calculated as a starting point, and you can make adjustments as needed. When you drop 1-2 pounds per week with little to no loss of strength, you've done it well. You're losing muscle when you lose a lot of strength, which indicates that you're not getting enough calories.

Here's how to figure out where to start:

- Consume 1.2 grams of protein daily for every pound of body weight.

- Consume 1 gram of carbs daily for every pound of body weight

- Consume 2 grams of healthy fat daily for every pound of body weight (1 gram daily for 5 pounds of body weight)

That is the initial step. This is what it might look like on a 140lb woman:

- 168 grams of protein daily.

- 140 grams of carbs daily.

- 28 grams of fat daily.

This equates to roughly 484 calories per day, which is a reasonable starting point for a lady weighing 140 pounds.

Your calculation is a little different if you are obese (body mass index of over 25% for males and 30% for women):

- 8 grams of protein daily for every pound of body weight.

- 7 grams of carbs daily for every pound of body weight.

- 3 grams of fat daily for every pound of body weight.

This is how it would appear for a woman weighing 175 pounds (notice that I'm rounding these figures down).

- 140 grams of protein per day.

- 120 grams of carbs per day

- 50 grams of fat per day

For a 175-pound woman, this equates to roughly 1,500 calories per day, which is a great spot to start weight loss.

Although most women find eating this much protein strange at first, consuming a lot of protein is actually essential for weight loss and for maintaining and growing muscle. Research, like the 2005 study from the University of Illinois, has demonstrated that high-protein diets help women maintain their muscle mass and, in an odd twist of logic, even lose more weight in the middle.

If you are having trouble maintaining this low fat level, you can adjust your diet by adding 20 grams more fat to your diet and cutting 50 grams less carbohydrates each day.

The Danger of Hidden Calorie Contents

Eating a lot of "hidden calorie contents" throughout the day and then wondering why they aren't losing weight is a massive, deadly diet trap that many people fall into. The following are examples of hidden calories that you may not be aware of:

- The two tablespoons of olive oil used to cook your chicken breast contains 240 calories.

- The two tablespoons of mayonnaise in your homemade chicken salad contains 200 calories.

- The three cubes of feta cheese on your salad contains 140 calories.

- The three tablespoons of cream in your coffee is made up of 80 calories.

- The two pats of butter with your toast has 70 calories.

The main cause of people's failure to see benefits from well-planned and calculated diets is hidden calorie contents. Simply put, they overeat, usually by going out to eat and getting what they believe to be low-calorie options from the menu.

As you can see, there isn't much room for mistake when dieting to lose weight because you will be operating on a daily 500–600 calorie deficit.
You won't lose much weight if you consume 400 hidden calories and, at the end of the day, only truly have a 100–200 calorie deficit. It's that easy. Although counting the number of tablespoons of ketchup you consume in a

day may seem excessive, you will undoubtedly see effects from your diet if you keep a tight eye on your caloric intake when trying to lose weight. You **WILL** get **LEAN**.

Making your own meal ensures that you know precisely what ingredients are in it and is the greatest method to eliminate hidden calorie contents (for most people, this simply entails making a lunch to take to work, as realists typically eat dinner at home).

Indications That Your Diet Is Incorrect Or Correct

You should evaluate the success of your diet after two to three weeks of adherence. But while determining whether or not your diet is working, there are other factors to take into account besides weight loss.

You ought to assess your development using the following standards:

Did your weight increase, decrease, or remain the same?

Do your clothes feel the same, tighter, or looser?

In the mirror, do you appear the same, fatter, or thinner?

How energetic are you? Do you feel exhausted, energized, or in the middle?

Your strength: is it increasing, decreasing, or remaining roughly the same?

Your sleep: do you struggle to fall asleep at night, are you always tired at the end of the day, or has nothing changed?

Let's take a quick look at each topic.

Weight

You're overeating if your weight is rising. You won't gain more muscle than the 1-2 pounds of fat you should be reducing each week, even if you're new to weightlifting.

If, after several weeks of dieting, your weight remains unchanged, you may be overeating, but it's also possible that you're simply gaining muscle to make up for the weight you lost from fat (you can tell which way you're doing this by looking in the mirror and your clothes, which we'll talk about).

If your weight is decreasing, that's a good indicator, but there are other things to make sure you're not undereating, which can lead to other issues (as you'll see in a moment).

Your clothes

It's a positive sign if your tops and jeans feel a little looser around the shoulders. You should consider yourself fortunate if your weight hasn't altered as well because you've reduced fat and gained muscle!

In Your Mirror

You should undoubtedly feel a difference after several weeks of dieting to lose weight, even though it can be difficult to notice changes in our bodies because we see them every day. You ought to appear more toned and less swollen.

If not, it's likely that neither your weight nor your sensation of looser clothes has altered. This is unmistakably evidence that you are still overeating.

If your weight hasn't changed despite your appearance in the mirror seeming smaller and your jeans fitting better, it's likely that you've gained muscle to make up for the lost fat or that your muscles are retaining more water. In any case, keep going as long as you're losing weight.

Your Energy Levels

Never should diets make you feel hungry or exhausted in an attempt to reduce weight. For the first week or two of the weight loss process, depending on how you ate before beginning the process, you might feel a bit hungry, but after that, you should feel comfortable all day long.

We all have days when we have more energy than others, but if you're experiencing more lows than usual, it's likely that you're not eating enough.

Your strength

Your strength ought to increase week after week if you're new to weight training and begin with dieting to lose weight. If not, this may be the result of improper nutrition, improper exercise, or improper rest.

Cutting carbohydrates might sometimes result in a slight loss of strength for seasoned weightlifters, although this loss shouldn't exceed 5%. You probably aren't eating enough if you see a 10% or more decline in strength.

Sleep

It's not always a terrible thing if you're exhausted by bedtime. When people begin training appropriately, this is typical.

The most crucial thing is to get a good night's sleep. You may be overtraining or undereating if you wake up more frequently at night, have a racing heartbeat, and exhibit anxiety or tossing and turning in bed.

Menstrual Cycle (Women)

You may not be able to determine this within the first three weeks of beginning a weight loss program, but you should be aware that undereating might cause hormonal imbalances if your cycle lengthens or becomes erratic.

However, if your cycles, which are typically erratic, start to become regular, this is most likely a positive indication that you're eating healthily.

In Summary;

Whether you think you may be overeating based on the above criteria, all you have to do is reduce your daily caloric intake by 200 and see whether that resolves the issue in the next two weeks. Just reduce your daily carbohydrate intake by 50 grams to cut these calories. Eat enough fats and proteins.

Whether you think you're not eating enough, increase your daily carb intake by 200 calories and observe whether that stabilizes your strength. It should.

It should be noted that for every 15 pounds lost, you should reduce your caloric intake by roughly 200. You should cut back on carbohydrates (50 grams per day) to offset these calories.

<u>Figuring Out What to Actually Eat and When</u>

Many individuals who are having trouble losing weight think they are eating little, but when they log their meals and look at the calories, they are consistently eating too much. Meal planning ahead of time allows you to ensure that you're eating the appropriate amount of food, which is an easy fix.

How then do you convert the calorie, protein, carb, and fat requirements into actual meals?
Easy! A food nutrition database, such as CalorieKing.com or Calorie count.about.com (my two favorites), is used to create meals.

It is crucial that you follow your workout diet plan precisely because, as you are aware, only a few hundred extra calories a day can completely negate your attempts to lose fat.

To figure this out, I suggest using a spreadsheet. The easiest approach to start is by making a list of all the meals for a whole day that you can make and eat. For every meal, make a list of every food's calories, protein, carbs, and fat and add up the amounts as you go. Adjust as necessary until you have enough food to match your daily needs for both macronutrients and calories.

Create stand-in meals that you can choose from whenever you want something different for breakfast, lunch, dinner, or other meals. I find that if I rotate my options every few days, I never get bored of any of them.

Now, let's work through a daily meal plan for a 150-pound man who wants to lose some weight. I'll use his nightly weightlifting as an example. I'll include a few meals from my cookbook, The Bodybuilding Meal Prep Cookbook. You can equally consult any other of my books.

Aim For Daily Carbs: 150grams
Aim For Daily Calories: 1,590
Aim For Daily Protein: 180grams Aim For Daily Fats: 30grams

Meal 1 (8:15am)
1 dish of scrambled veggies with cheese and eggs
273 calories
32 grams of protein
8 grams of carbs
9 grams of fat

Meal 2 (10:30am)
1 cup of low-fat cottage cheese
1 medium orange
265 calories

30 grams of protein
16 grams of carbs
4 grams of fat

Meal 3 (12:30pm)
1 dish of Quick &Easy Protein Salad
272 calories
24 grams of protein
31 grams of carbs
5 grams of fat

Meal 4 (3:30pm)
1 Strawberry Banana Protein Bar
199 calories
22 grams of protein
16 grams of carbs
5 grams of fat

Meal 5 (pre-workout 5:30pm)
1 scoop of protein powder in water
1 medium orange
190 calories
30 grams of protein
16 grams of carbs
Zero fat

Meal 6 (post-workout 7:00pm)
1 dish of Graham-Coated Tilapia
1 apple
320 calories
25 grams of protein
35 grams of carbs
10 grams of fat

Meal 7 (10:30pm)

20 grams of casein or egg protein
80 calories
20 grams of protein
Zero grams of carbs
1 gram of fat

Summary

Our 150-pound friend can start losing weight with this meal plan, which has 1,599 calories, 183 grams of protein, 122 grams of (carbs) carbohydrates, and 34 grams of fat.

Keep in mind that the figures you compute are targets; you don't need to rack your brains attempting to balance meals or components to reach them precisely or within a very narrow range.

DIETING MAINTENANCE

As soon as you're satisfied with your level of leanness and want to gradually strengthen and build muscle without gaining any more fat, you should follow a diet.

Now, "maintaining" does not mean "staying the same."Most individuals usually want to enhance the shape or appearance of specific parts of their bodies, so I believe your monthly objective should be to get at least a bit stronger. Always aim to develop and set goals. Because things usually either grow better or worse, don't try to stay the same.

Calculating Your Maintenance Diet

Here's how you choose where to start:
- Consume one gram of protein daily for every pound of body weight.
- Consume 1.5 grams of carbohydrates daily per pound of body weight.
- Consume 1 gram of good fats for every 4 pounds of body weight each day.

That is the initial step. If a person weighed 130 pounds, it would appear like this:

- 130 grams of protein day
- 195 grams of carbohydrates daily
- 32 grams of fat day

That equates to roughly 1,600 calories a day, which ought to be sufficient to build muscle and strength gradually without gaining any additional fat.

<u>General Rules For Maintaining</u>

Make a daily eating plan and follow it religiously. Don't worry if you're 50–100 calories over your goal.

Of course, you can arrange a variety, but you should be aware of exactly what you put into your body on a daily basis.

You don't need to worry about refeeding because your carbohydrate intake is sufficient, and you may still indulge once or twice a week.

Enjoy a post-workout meal that contains at least 30% of your daily carbohydrates, but feel free to consume more if you'd like.

Keep in mind that loading up on carbohydrates is ideal during the "window" following exercise.

<u>Indications That Your Diet Is Incorrect Or Correct</u>

The same standards used to evaluate your weight reduction diet should also be used to assess your progress.

Compared to dieting to lose weight, keeping your current weight is not as good a measure of your progress. Every week, you can gain a little muscle and shed a little fat, but your weight should essentially remain constant. Your weight may increase if you gain a little muscle but remain fat-free, or it may decrease if you lose a little muscle or fat because of insufficient food intake.

Every week, you should be growing a little stronger and seeing small positive changes in the way your clothes fit. If, after a few weeks of sticking to your maintenance diet, your jeans are getting tighter and you look flabbier, you are probably eating too much. You should also be sleeping well and have good energy levels. If neither of these things are happening, you may be eating too little or too much of the wrong kinds of food (too many trans fats or high-GI carbohydrates, for example).

After a few weeks of observation, if you think you're eating too much, subtract 200 calories from your daily goal by consuming 50 grams less carbohydrates. Cut deeper if it doesn't.

Increase your daily calorie intake by 200 if you think you're not eating enough. Keep in mind that fats have 9 calories per gram and carbohydrates have 4.

THE COMPOSITION OF YOUR BODY IS MORE IMPORTANT THAN BODY WEIGHT

Some people may be a little perplexed by their progress on the Become Thinner Leaner Stronger program because they have been so thoroughly taught to value their weight above everything else.

People frequently begin this regimen and, unless they are extremely slim (15% body fat or less), actually gain muscle while reducing fat. Although it may not seem like much is changing on the scale, they are definitely making improvement when they observe their actions in the gym and in the mirror.

My acquaintance who has been training for the past 10 months is a perfect illustration of this. He weighed a little over 220 pounds and had roughly 23% body fat when he began. His strength had almost doubled in the first three months of training, and for the first time in his life, he had visible muscle. However, he had lost twenty pounds since the beginning of his training, which can be quite upsetting for men like us who associate strength and size with increased weight. Naturally, he lost all of this fat—his body fat percentage was 14%.

Seven months later, he has put on almost twenty pounds of muscle, bringing his weight back to where it was before he began, but many are amazed at the drastic change in his body composition.

If your weight isn't changing but your power is increasing, your muscles are visibly growing tighter, and you're shedding fat, don't worry if you're not already fit and thin. Pay attention to the scale, but ultimately let your mirror and weights speak for you.

IN SUMMARY

Although I realize it's a lot to process at once, I have excellent news. Everything you'll ever need to know about dieting has just been imparted to you. If you only apply the advice in the last few chapters, you won't ever again struggle to grow muscle or lose fat. Please feel free to go back and read this section of the book several times to ensure that everything truly clicks.

Now let's talk about training and how to get the most of our daily workouts.

Chapter 18

BECOME THINNER LEANER STRONGER TRAINING FORMULA

There are several similar training systems that are advertised in periodicals and infomercials. They want you to perform a lot of repetitions using a variety of machines and possibly some light free weights. Dumbbells are typically used in free weight exercises, which target specific muscles such the shoulders, triceps, and biceps.

There are far better ways to spend your time and energy than on this kind of exercise, even though it is still better than nothing.

Strangely, the reason why machines have become a mainstay in gyms is not their effectiveness, but rather their appeal. They don't appear to be as menacing as iron bars and hunks. They're simpler to work with and, in certain situations, pose less danger of harm.

While some machines are helpful, like the cable setup, most are not as effective as exercises using dumbbells and barbells in building larger, more toned muscles. For this reason, free weights rather than machines will be the main focus of the *Become Thinner Leaner Stronger* workout program.

When using free weights, individuals typically perform isolated exercises. This kind of exercise originated in the men's bodybuilding community, where some males dedicate hours of their daily lives to the gym, carefully shaping every muscle fiber in their bodies in preparation for competitions or to use their physical attractiveness as a tool to attract women. Workouts based on this type of training are obviously not the best for ladies who wish to appear slender and sporty.

The foundation of the *Become Thinner Leaner Stronger* program consists of compound movements such as the Military Press, Bench Press, Deadlift,

Squat, and many more. When it comes to time and effort, these are the workouts that provide the greatest overall strengthening and conditioning for the entire body.

The *Become Thinner Leaner Stronger* weight training method uses the following formula:

$$1\text{--}2 \mid 8\text{--}10 \mid 12 \mid 1\text{--}2 \mid 45\text{--}60 \mid 5\text{--}7 \mid 8\text{--}10$$

No, you don't need to crack a secret code to access that. Let's examine each component of this formula separately.

1–2

EACH DAY, TRAIN 1 – 2 MAJOR MUSCLE GROUPS

During each workout (per day), you will focus on exercising one or two primary muscle groups. You will do three different types of workouts: one that targets only one major muscle group (like the legs or chest), one that targets one major group plus one minor group (like the back and abs), or one that targets two minor groups (like the triceps and biceps).

Become Thinner Leaner Stronger is organized for two reasons. First of all, two major muscle groups cannot be adequately trained in an hour or less of exercise (you will soon discover why 45 to 60 minutes is the ideal length for your training sessions). The psychological explanation is the second. You can train a major muscle group with 100% focus and intensity if you train it just once a day.

8–10

PERFORM NEARLY ALL EXERCISES IN SETS OF 8–10 REPS.

For the most part, you'll be performing 8–10 repetitions every set of exercises (the exception being ab training, where you should choose a weight that allows you to perform 15–20 reps).

What does "8–10 reps" mean? This means that you should utilize weights that are neither too light nor too heavy to prevent you from performing more than eight repetitions. The weight is too heavy if you find that an activity requires you to perform at least 8 repetitions; on the other hand, if you find that you can perform more than 10 reps, the weight is too light.

You should increase the weight in your following set (5 pounds for dumbbell exercises and 10 pounds for barbell exercises) once you can do a set of 10 repetitions with flawless form. After that, you should be able to do 8 repetitions on your subsequent set, and over the ensuing weeks, you can increase your strength. If you can't get at least 8 repetitions on your next set, decrease to a 5-pound increase if an increase of 10 pounds seems excessive.

You've probably never done this kind of training before because most weightlifting regimens require you to use incredibly light weights. But as you are now aware, there is very little that this type of training can do to increase your strength, muscle mass, or definition. However, you can significantly increase your strength as well as the shape and tone of your muscles by using weights that will only allow you to perform 8–10 repetitions. You can also achieve this by gradually increasing the weights you use over time.

Be prepared for a challenge, then. Prepare to exert yourself. Exercise ought to feel laborious. Every set doesn't have to end in complete failure (the point at which you can't possibly perform another rep no matter how hard you try), but your last reps should be difficult without compromising form.

12

PERFORM 12 WORKING SETS PER MUSCLE GROUP

Your workouts will consist of 12 "working" sets per muscle group trained. A working set is your challenging, 8– 10 reps, muscle-building set, as opposed to a warm-up set, which we'll soon go over.

Regardless of which exercises you do, you'll never do more than 12 sets for any individual muscle group.

This might be a shock to some. All too often I see people pounding away on a muscle group, doing 20, 25, or even 30 sets of lifting. This is overtraining, and it's not only a huge waste of time but a huge waste of muscle—both potential and existing. The body can't effectively repair that much damage to the muscle fibers, and the result can actually be shrinkage.

12 working sets is the sweet spot for total training volume for each muscle group given the weights you'll be handling. By doing 12 working sets per muscle group, you not only fully and deeply stimulate the muscles you're training, but you can keep your workouts in the ideal time frame of 45–60 minutes.

1–2

REST 1–2 MINUTES IN BETWEEN SETS

Numerous physiological processes occur as you lift weights in order to complete the activity. A muscle needs oxygen, cellular energy, specific chemical reactions, and numerous other biochemical activities in order to contract. You exhaust your muscles' ability to contract forcefully with each repetition.

You can only repeat this process to the point where you reach the ideal level of muscular overload necessary to force and promote new growth if you give yourself adequate time to recuperate between sets. Essentially, the goal of taking a break in between sets is to prime your muscles for the next set's maximal weightlifting.

The recuperation interval between sets should be between one and two minutes. This duration enables your muscles to fully recover from the previous session by refueling their energy reserves and eliminating any undesirable chemical residue.

There are days when you'll feel more energised and recover more quickly, and days when you'll feel a little slower. It's crucial that you allow yourself ample rest periods in between sets so that you can lift the most weight possible throughout each set. It's fine if you require the entire two minutes; if you only need one, that's also acceptable.

But don't make rest periods last longer than five or six minutes. This destroys intensity and makes the workout drag out. The question isn't whether you **WANT** to do the next set or not; rather, it's if you feel like you have the energy to perform another set and your body's pulse rate has decreased since the last set.

<u>45–60</u>

TRAIN FOR ABOUT 45–60 MINUTES

Something is amiss if your workouts are taking more than an hour. Every *Become Thinner Leaner Stronger* exercise should take you no more than 45 minutes to complete, and never more than an hour. (Resting a little longer on some days is necessary; this takes time, as does completing ab exercises.)

The typical cause of workouts lasting longer than ninety minutes is that individuals tend to neglect their rest periods, engaging in conversation with friends during the six, seven, or even ten-minute breaks between sets.

Extended exercises are detrimental in two aspects. First of all, it's challenging to keep up a sustained level of mental and physical exertion for an hour and a half (particularly if you're taking five minutes to relax in between sets). Second, your body releases hormones such as cortisol, growth hormone, and testosterone when you exercise. After roughly an hour of exercise, all three of these hormones peak, and your cortisol keeps rising while your growth hormone and testosterone start to decline. Your body becomes more catabolic the higher your cortisol levels. Overtraining symptoms arise when training in this state for longer than necessary. You should stop exercise in around 60 minutes or less to allow your cortisol levels, testosterone, and growth hormone levels to drop and maintain anabolism.

The fact that it's good to not have to spend a lot of time in the gym every day is another advantage of shorter workouts. Almost anyone can find out how to change their body in around an hour, out of 35 days a week.

5-7

ONE TRAINING PER MUSCLE GROUP EVERY 5-7 DAYS
The duration of rest between training sessions is a critical factor in determining the amount of muscular growth (or lack thereof) in a certain muscle type. Recall that while overloading your muscles causes them to grow, the actual growth happens outside of the gym when your body changes the muscle to make it stronger and more resilient to overloads in the future.

All of the above strategies to help you achieve the body you desire depend on your ability to recover. No matter how closely you adhere to the rest of this training protocol, you will not make significant progress if you don't give your body enough time to recover from a workout before overloading the same muscles again. If you carry on in this manner for an extended period of time, you will become weaker and flabby, your energy and appetite will both decline, and you won't have any desire to train.

Research has indicated that following weight training, the body needs a full two to five days to recover damaged muscles. This is felt by humans as "delayed onset muscle soreness," or DOMs, a reduction in inflammation and pain in the muscles.

How long our bodies require to recover now depends on a variety of factors, including our genetics, level of general fitness, and the intensity and duration of our workouts (i.e., how hard we train and how many sets we complete).

I'm going to offer you 5–7 days to assure full recovery from the *Become Thinner Leaner Stronger* routines, even though some people will be done in 3–4 days. Trying to fit in an extra leg session each week is not worth the danger of overtraining.

8–10

AVOID TRAINING FOR A WEEK EVERY 8–10 WEEKS.

This kind of lifting might be very difficult. It weighs a much. It's quite strong. It will hurt your muscles. You'll need to adjust your joints.

Additionally, research indicates that the central nervous system need 7–14 days to fully recuperate from the strains associated with weightlifting. Training three to five days a week will gradually overwhelm your Central Nervous System (CNS), necessitating occasional full rest periods.

Every few months, taking a week off from training is actually a crucial component of general healing and restoration. Your body need a break after 8–10 weeks of training in order to fully recover, and you will physically experience this (by week 8 or 9, don't be shocked if you feel weak, short on energy, and uninterested in training—all signs of overtraining starting to manifest).

Don't worry about gaining weight or becoming weaker during your week off. It is not going to occur. On the other hand, your body might enter a hyper-anabolic condition and you can return substantially stronger if you eat well during your week off.

One further crucial aspect of your week off is that you should avoid engaging in any intense physical activity (such as weightlifting or intense cardio) during the week. Being a slug doesn't have to happen, but you shouldn't put your body through needless stress.

Now, I suggest that you attempt a "Reduce-load Week" if, following your initial few weeks off, you discover that you return feeling weaker and fatigued. I carry this out.

I used to entirely rest for one week around every two months, but my body didn't seem to appreciate it. My friends would usually return stronger than me. My current method functions far better.

Whenever I go to the gym, I do 6–9 light sets with 40–50% of my usual weight instead of my usual heavylifting routine, and I never fail. I perform 8–10 repetitions every set, just enough to generate a slight pump. Keep in mind that your body requires time to regulate its Central Nervous System (CNS), so avoid putting it under excessive stress.

All I want to do is enhance protein synthesis and recovery by increasing blood flow (and nutrients) to the muscles, as studies have demonstrated.

I advise you to try weeks of total rest during the first 6–9 months of this regimen. Try the "Reduce-load Week" if, after attempting a few fullest weeks, your body still doesn't feel right or if you return weakened. I believe you will enjoy it.

CARDIO

Many criticize cardiac exercise just because they dislike it. I know this because I was one of them once.

Cardio can help you gain (and keep) more muscle in three main ways. They are listed in the following order:

1. It enhances muscle recuperation by augmenting blood circulation to the muscles.

2. It helps you reduce the amount of fat stored by enhancing your body's metabolic reactions to food.

3. Maintaining your conditioning helps your body adjust more smoothly to the change from "bulking" to "cutting."

However, excessive cardio can hinder your progress by overtraining you and drastically decreasing your calorie surplus. However, if you only adhere to my suggestions, this should not present any problems for you.

AFTER LIFTING OR BEFORE LIFTING IS CARDIO BEST? NOT ONE!

Gains in strength and muscle can be severely impeded by cardiac exercise immediately before or after weightlifting. Why?

In 2009, RMIT University researchers who worked with highly skilled athletes discovered that "combining resistance exercise and cardio in the same session may disrupt genes for anabolism." Simply put, scientists discovered that sending "mixed signals" to the muscles when endurance and resistance exercise are combined.

Anabolic hormones including MGF and IGF-1 were inhibited by cardio prior to strength training, while muscle tissue breakdown was elevated following resistance training.

Numerous more research, including those from the University of Jyvaskyla (Finland), the Waikato Institute of Technology, and the Children's National Medical Center, reached the same conclusions: exercising for strength and endurance at the same time hinders progress in both areas. It is significantly better to train only for strength or endurance during a workout.

Prior to lifting weights, cardio depletes your energy and makes it more difficult to exercise hard, which prevents the building of new muscle.

How then do you do it correctly?

THE THREE CARDIOVASCULAR COMMANDMENTS

Here's how to keep cardio from interfering with your muscle growth, whether you're doing it for health reasons, just because you enjoy it, or to help lose fat.

1. Do cardio 3–5 times a week.

According to studies, three aerobic workouts a week are sufficient to enhance both muscular growth and cardiovascular health. Therefore, I advise you to do cardio at least three days a week, even if you're just sustaining.

Most believe that exercising is essential to reaching the 15% and below "super lean" category since there's a limit to how many calories you can cut without losing muscle and strength. For example, I have to do cardio to drop below 10% because I can't reduce my calorie intake any farther without experiencing severe discomfort.

However, some folks are not worth bothering. They only control their caloric intake to get the desired level of leanness. It basically comes down to individual physiology and genetics. When you genuinely diet to lose weight, you'll discover which category you fit into, but in order to speed up your fat loss, aim to undertake cardio three to five times a week.

2. Spend 20 to 30 minutes per session doing cardio-focused high-intensity interval training (HIIT).

Long, low-intensity cardio workouts are unsuccessful at assisting with fat loss since they typically have a detrimental effect on muscle growth and burn comparatively little calories.

However, compared to low-intensity, steady-state cardio, shorter, high-intensity sessions not only result in less muscle breakdown but also burn more calories and promote greater fat loss (see studies from Laval University, East Tennessee State University, Baylor College of Medicine, and the University of New South Wales).

For this reason, I advise using HIIT for all cardio and keeping your workouts between 20 and 30 minutes. This is how it operates:

- A two- to three-minute low-intensity warm-up precedes your workout.

- After that, you exert all of your energy for 30 to 60 seconds, depending on your experience level with HIIT. 30-second intervals should be sufficient for beginners, but you should aim to complete 60-second intervals as well.

- Then, for the same amount of time as your high-intensity interval, you reduce it to a low-intensity recovery phase. Once more, you might need to make this rest period 1.5–2 times longer than your high intensity interval if you're new to HIIT. You're not prepared to return to the high-intensity level if you're still having trouble breathing and your heart rate is elevated.

- For twenty to thirty minutes, you repeat this cycle of all-out and recuperation intervals.

- You cool down for two to three minutes at a low effort.

You can incorporate the HIIT method into any regular cardio exercise. You can complete the task by using the recumbent bike or elliptical trainer, or you can go outside and run or walk.

3. Give yourself a few hours between your weightlifting and cardio workouts.

You already understand the benefits of separating your aerobic and weight training, but regrettably, the research did not suggest a duration of time between them.

After experimenting with a variety of intervals, I've discovered that at least 23 hours works well. In theory, it is generally preferable to wait longer. I currently work out with weights for roughly 14 hours after cardio because I work out early in the morning and finish my cardio workout around 9:30 pm.

I advise performing your cardio after weightlifting, never before, and no more than 20 to 30 minutes of high-intensity interval training (HIIT) if you are unable to separate the two exercises. Although that's not the best arrangement, your strength gains won't be undone by it.

LIFTING WEIGHTS WHILE GOING ON A DIET TO REDUCE WEIGHT

The worst piece of advice when it comes to getting thin is probably to train with light weights in order to get "really cut." Ninety percent of this is incorrect. It is not true that lighter weights burn more fat than bigger weights. They fail to "bring out definition in a real way." You don't become toned by them. Really, they are just a huge waste of time.

When you're on a diet to lose weight, training hard is **EXTRA** crucial since it will help you keep your muscle because you'll be forcing your body to continue overloading it.

Don't be shocked if you really build some strength and muscle while reducing weight if you stick to a strict diet and exercise regimen. (If you tell your buddies that you lift weights, they will be envious!)

FINAL SENTENCE

These are the main principles of the weight training program Become Thinner Leaner Stronger. It's likely that this is how you've always lifted, and if so, you should be thrilled about it.

You'll soon be able to enjoy consistent, obvious muscular growth—without bulking up—by engaging in relatively quick, intense workouts that yield outcomes that other people can only imagine.

Chapter 19

MEET YOUR MAKERS: FIVE EXERCISES THAT BUILDS GREAT BODIES

Achieving a great physique involves a balanced approach to fitness. Five key exercises that contribute to building a strong and impressive body include squats, deadlifts, bench presses, pull-ups, and planks. Each targets multiple muscle groups, fostering overall strength and muscle development. Incorporating these exercises into a well-rounded workout routine can lead to noticeable improvements in both strength and aesthetics.

The majority of individuals train incorrectly.

They will claim that it's "better for their shoulders" if they stop their bench presses six inches or higher over their chest. Because they "don't want to stress their knees," they'll load up a lot of plates, stoop down a foot or two, then stand backup. When performing Deadlifts, they will hunch their backs to "really go heavy," and at the top, they will heavily arch their lower backs to "really get a squeeze."

Inadequate form not only impedes progress, but it also leaves room for harm. The Bench Press is a heavy, half-rep exercise that puts undue strain on your shoulders. In actuality, half-squats are detrimental to your knees, while doing a full range of motion with reasonable weights improves them. A severe injury is just waiting to happen when deadlifting involves hunched repetitions and excessive back arching.

Conversely, if you lift with complete awareness of form and throughout your range of motion, you will experience complete muscular development, consistent increases, and avoidable aches and problems.

Now, let's review correct form for a few of the main exercises that you will perform throughout this program.

THE SQUAT

I have the utmost respect for anyone in the gym who can properly squat, no matter what kind of weight they use.

Sadly, hardly many individuals truly get it properly. Of course, performing half reps—that is, not lowering the body until the hips are lower than the knees—is the most frequent mistake. Proper squats actually develop the muscles that support the knees and prevent damage, while shallow squats cause all sorts of knee problems, especially when done with greater weights.

Because it works wonders for your entire body, the squat is a safe and very effective workout that you will enjoy to execute when done well.

You may scream, cry, or groan if you squat properly and with a lot of weight—heavy for you—but you generally won't hurt yourself.

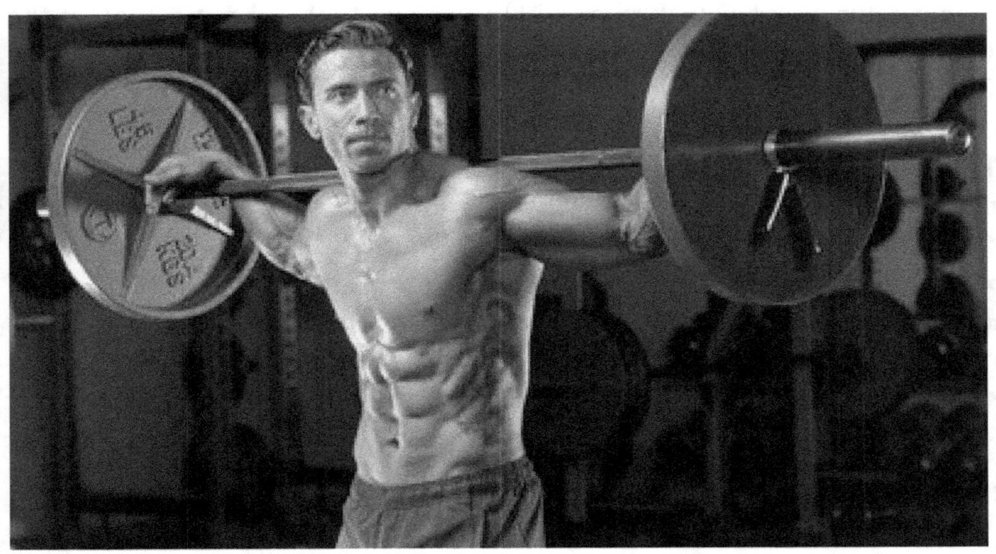

Squatting is regarded by many as the "King of Exercises" and is among the most effective, if not the greatest, exercises available. Additionally, it is among the hardest to learn. If you are unfamiliar with this exercise, please practice with an empty bar or broomstick for multiple training sessions (you can work on the leg press further if necessary). It's critical to perfect your form while the weights are still light. When you use large weights, your little mistakes with tiny weights will become HUGE mistakes. The squat has gotten a lot of negative publicity in the media, although this criticism mostly stems from poor form rather than the workout itself. We'll highlight potential red flags and perhaps provide advice on how to avoid them.

First Thing First

Appropriate trunk position should be discussed before foot position or stance width. Assume that the meanest, ugliest sergeant in history has just yelled at you, "TEN-HUT!" Naturally, you would raise yourself up and tuck your shoulders back. This is how the spine should be positioned for a squat. That is, you have a little arch in your lower back, your head pulled back, and your chest elevated. You should never glance down or bend down at the low back during a squat. It goes without saying that you must bend at the hips (more on that later). Neither of you should look up. Okay, so you understand that?

The ideal place to perform squats these days is in a power rack or cage, which is a big rectangular rack with cross-drilled holes. This allows you to modify the pins so that, in the event that you need to bale, you can safely lower the bar. Just below the depth you plan to go, set the pins. Additionally, they provide as a visual signal for depth and if you move crookedly up or down. Approximately where your nipple is, place the J hooks or posts that hold the bar for you to get beneath. To check whether it is at the proper height, try unracking it once. There should be a knurled section in the center of the bar; if not, go to another bar or gym.

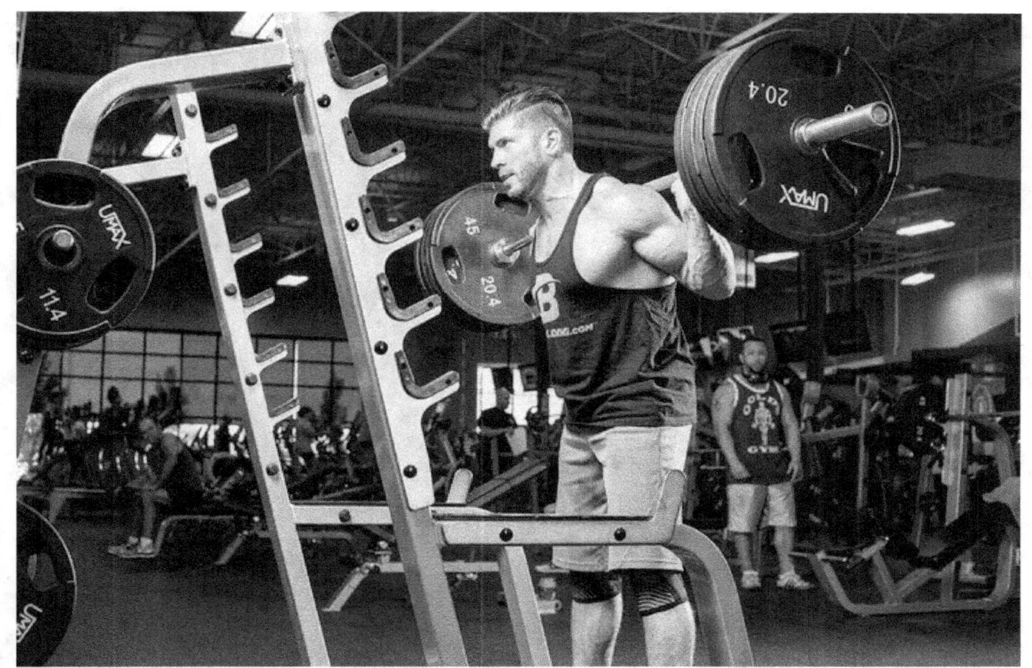

Barbell Squat

Under the bar, a lot of folks utilize towels or padding. A few people, myself included, believe that this causes some instability since the weight is "teeter tottering" on a little spot on your back. If the bar is painful, you should either get a Manta Ray, add additional trapezius mass, or accept it as a necessary component of the exercise and move the bar a little further down your back, just above or below the sharp ridge on your scapula (shoulder blade). Although it doesn't suit everyone well, the Ray aids in distributing the weight over the shoulder.

Proceed to the bar now. Unless you are performing the wide-grip shoulder breaker version, place your hands approximately the breadth of a bench press, and make sure you are even on the bar before unracking. Inhale deeply, move beneath the bar, and unrack it. According to Fred Hatfield, the majority of squat accidents happen during the back up. On the descent, just take as many steps as necessary to clear the posts or j-hooks. Even during the unracking and back up, keep in mind the "soldier position".

Spread your feet shoulder-width apart or a little more apart. Consider how a thread hanging from the ceiling can strike your ankle and rub against your medial delt.

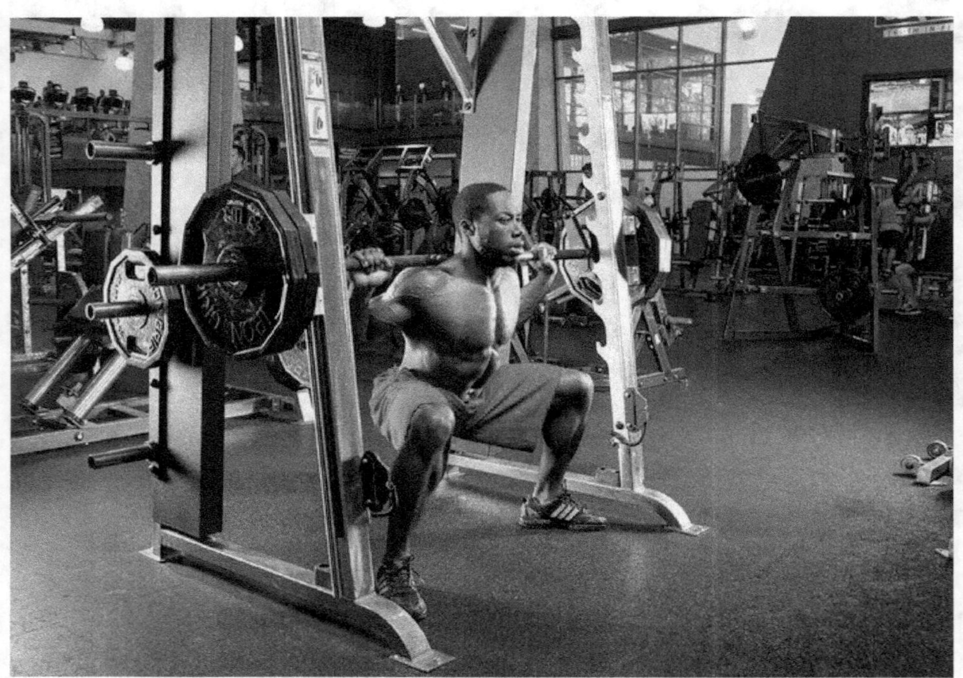

Utilize the "practice" sessions to determine your ideal width. You might say that a lot of powerlifters have a wide stance when they squat, and as a group, they are quite strong. I completely concur, but I'll add mention that because you're working through a greater range of motion, the traditional squat is probably more effective. If you'd like, learn the variations after mastering this method. Once the breadth is appropriate, extend your feet to a roughly 45-degree angle. Adapt the width as necessary. You are now prepared to squat.

Inhale deeply, tense your abdomen, and lower yourself down. Instead of falling straight down, it should seem like you are reclining on a chair behind you. Make sure your knees are parallel to your feet. **AVOID LETTING YOUR KNEES BOW DURING THE LIFT!** I did this and now have a Grade 1 MCL sprain in my knee. To avoid doing this, keep the load modest enough and increase gradually. It's common knowledge to aim to maintain your shin at a 90-degree angle to the floor. Few people can accomplish this with the conventional stance squat; only those using the wide-stance variation can. Try not to extend your knees past your toes. Adjust the width as necessary. Most people should drop until their thighs are parallel to the floor. In fact, they should. Actually, this is rather low. Most individuals can't, and it might be best to stop slightly above the parallel for them.

Keep trying until you get parallel. Furthermore, you have to bend at the hips (not the spine, of course) in order to become even somewhat parallel. Still, you ought to be standing rather than stooping at all times. There are two ways to find your shin/back position and depth: either have someone skilled and aware watch you from the side, or use a camera that is positioned to the side and close enough to pick up every aspect. Once you have reached the lowest place, instantly reverse your orientation and drive upward, avoiding bouncing at the bottom. During the climb, make a concerted effort to pull your hip extension (back up).

This is described by Brooks Kubik as "as if a giant gorilla had a hold of your ass and your shoulder and was trying to straighten you out." Resuming your upright position, inhale deeply (or deeply) and then lower yourself once more. In between reps, keep in mind the soldier position as well. Give every rep a little lift of its own. Make every one of them matter, even during your warm-ups. You're more likely to keep your form during the work sets if you keep it up during your warm-ups.

Belts Or Knee Wraps

Is it better to use knee wraps or a belt? By raising intra-abdominal pressure, the former serves to support the spine, whereas the latter only raises the weight. Avoid both, particularly if you are just starting out with the squat. Instead of using outside assistance as a brace, use your abdomen. Except for the powerlifter who wants a bigger max, the knee wraps are useless. When used repeatedly, they might possibly be harmful or prevent the development of structures surrounding the knee.

Squats hurt! That's the major reason the power rack collects dust while there's a wait for the angled leg press! Whether it's the skinny newbie utilizing the "big wheels" on both sides for the first time or the legitimate 600+ squatter stepping under a bar that's already bent, it makes no difference. When performing this activity, they both experience minor pain. Acquire the ability to cope with it!

The hardest workouts are also the most fruitful. That is a reality. You may scream, cry, throw up, or even pass out if you squat properly and with a lot of weight—heavy for you—but you won't likely be hurt and you'll get closer to your objectives. Develop an aggressive mindset and give the task at hand your whole concentration. Wishing you success and joy in your training!

THE DEADLIFT

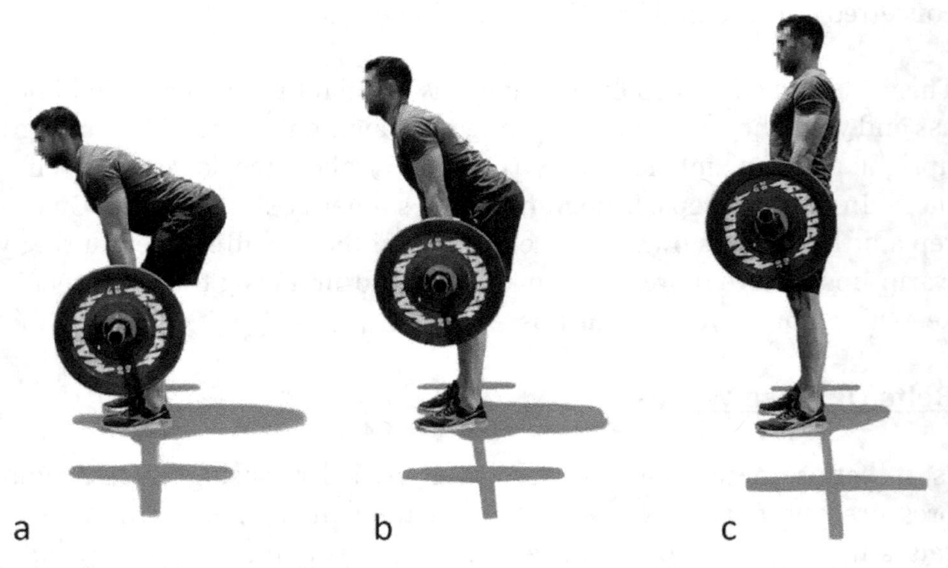

a   b   c

The deadlift is a compound weightlifting exercise that targets multiple muscle groups, including the lower back, glutes, hamstrings, and core. It involves lifting a loaded barbell from the ground to a standing position, with the lifter's hips and knees fully extended.

There are various deadlift variations, such as conventional, sumo, and Romanian deadlifts, each emphasizing different aspects of muscle engagement and targeting specific areas. Proper form is crucial to prevent injury, with key points including a flat back, engaged core, and proper hip hinge.

Deadlifts are renowned for their effectiveness in building overall strength and muscle mass. They stimulate the posterior chain, enhance grip strength, and promote functional fitness. Due to their intensity, it's essential to progressively increase weights and incorporate adequate rest between sessions to allow for recovery.

While deadlifts offer numerous benefits, individuals with existing back issues or injuries should exercise caution and may need modifications. As with any exercise, consulting a fitness professional or healthcare provider is advisable before incorporating deadlifts into a workout routine.

THE BENCH PRESS

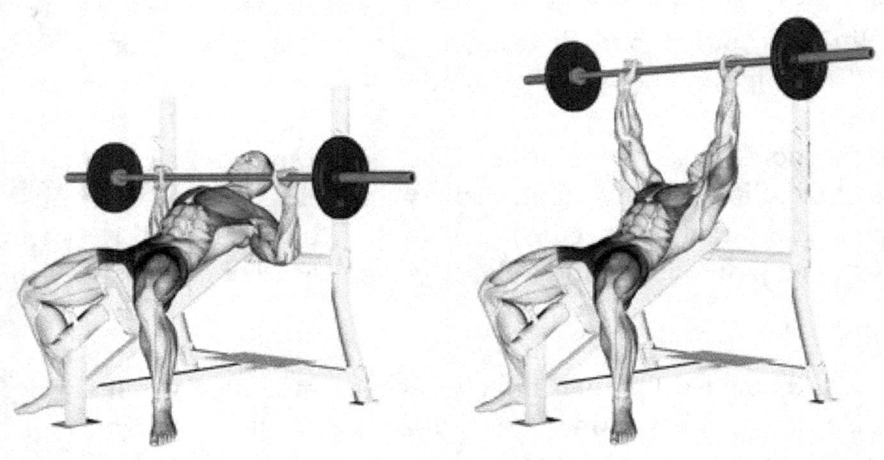

The bench press is a popular strength training exercise that primarily targets the chest, shoulders, and triceps. It involves lying on a bench and lifting a barbell loaded with weights. It's a fundamental exercise in many strength training programs.

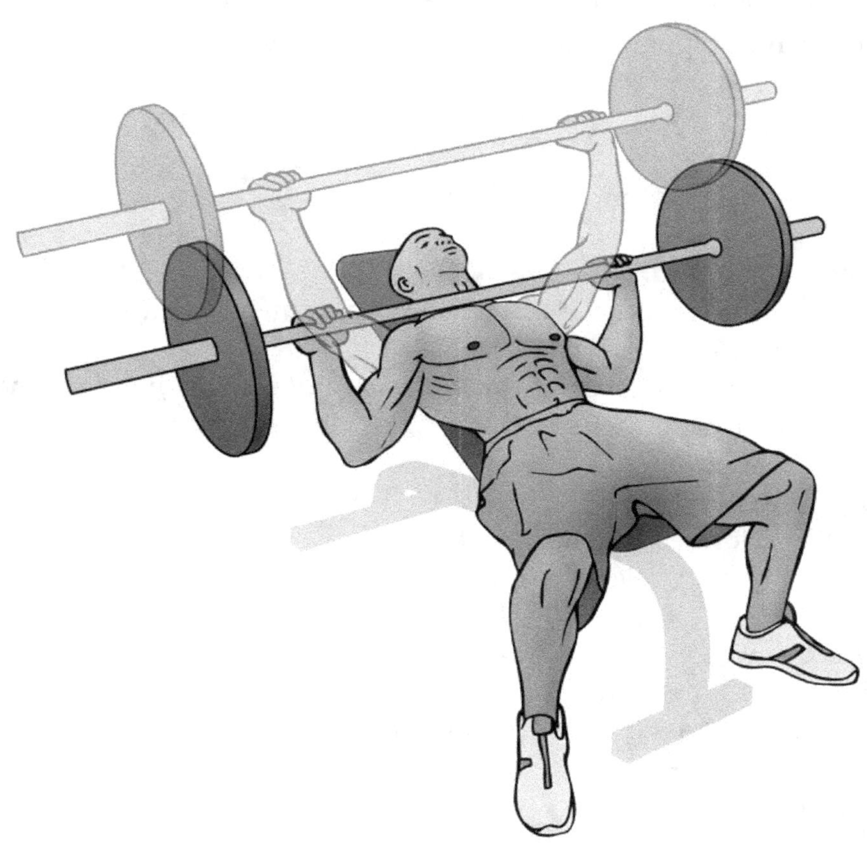

Description

With your feet flat on the ground and little wider than shoulder-width apart, take a seat on an inclined bench. Make sure your eyes are level with the bar as you lie down, and check up as often as necessary to adjust.

- Reach for the bar. Your hands should be positioned on the bar on each side, about five inches outside of your head. Take a deep breath just before you raise.

- Lift the weight off the rack, then bring it toward your chest in a two-second count, stopping two inches from your chest (never bounce!).

- Exhale upward as you raise the weight to your maximum extension.

Key points about the bench press include:

1. **Muscles Targeted:**
- Primary: Pectoralis major (chest muscles), anterior deltoids (front shoulder muscles), triceps brachii.
- Secondary: Latissimus dorsi (back muscles), serratus anterior, and various stabilizing muscles.

2. **Equipment:**
- Typically performed on a flat bench.
- Involves a barbell, weights, and a rack for support.

3. **Variations:**
- Incline Bench Press: Targets upper chest.
- Decline Bench Press: Focuses on lower chest.
- Dumbbell Bench Press: Uses dumbbells for more independent arm movement.

4. **Execution:**
- Lie on your back, grip the barbell slightly wider than shoulder-width apart.
- Lower the barbell to your chest and then press it back up.
- Maintain proper form, including a stable back and controlled movement.

5. **Benefits:**
- Builds upper body strength and muscle mass.
- Enhances pushing power.
- Engages multiple muscle groups.

6. Safety Tips:

- Use a spotter, especially when lifting heavy weights.
- Warm up adequately to prevent injuries.
- Maintain proper form to avoid strain on joints.

7. Training Program:

- Often included in strength training and powerlifting routines.
- Incorporate progressive overload by gradually increasing weights.

8. Common Mistakes:

- Arching the back excessively.
- Bouncing the bar off the chest.
- Neglecting proper warm-up.

9. Records and Competitions:

- Bench press is a standard in powerlifting competitions.
- Various weight classes and age divisions exist.

10. Cautions:

- Individuals with shoulder or back issues should exercise caution.
- Ensure the equipment is properly set up.

11. Incorporation in Fitness Programs:

- Suitable for both beginners and advanced lifters.
- Often part of a comprehensive upper body workout routine.

Remember, proper form is crucial to prevent injuries and maximize the effectiveness of the exercise. Consult with a fitness professional or healthcare provider if you have any concerns or pre-existing conditions.

THE PULL-UPS

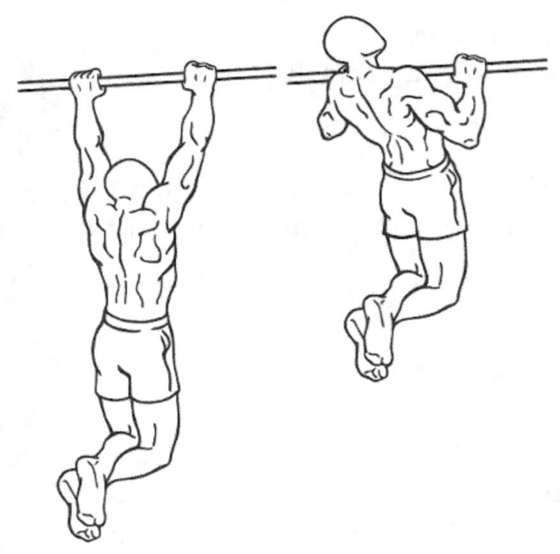

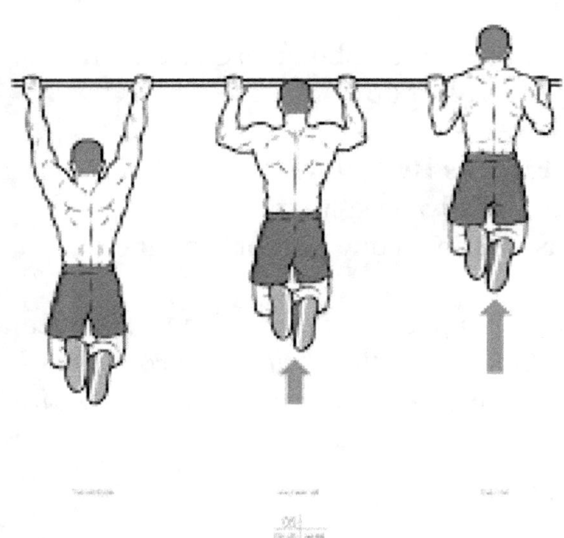

Pull-ups focus on targeting specific muscle groups, including the latissimus dorsi, biceps, and upper back. To optimize gains, ensure a full range of motion, control your descent, and vary grip positions like wide and narrow to engage different muscles. Gradually increase resistance for progressive overload and incorporate pull-up variations for a well-rounded upper body workout.

Pull-ups are a compound exercise primarily targeting the upper back, lats, and biceps. Incorporating pull-ups into your routine can enhance overall upper body strength and muscle development. To optimize bodybuilding pull-ups:

1. **Grip Variations**: Experiment with wide, narrow, and neutral grips to target different muscle groups. Wide grips emphasize the outer lats, while a narrow grip engages the inner back and biceps.

2. **Proper Form**: Maintain a controlled and smooth movement throughout the exercise. Focus on pulling with your back muscles, not just relying on arm strength. Ensure a full range of motion, lowering your body until your arms are fully extended.

3. **Scapular Retraction**: Emphasize scapular retraction by pulling your shoulder blades together at the bottom of each rep. This maximizes back engagement and muscle contraction.

4. **Weighted Pull-Ups**: Progress by adding weight gradually using a weight belt or a weighted vest. This increases resistance, promoting muscle growth and strength development.

5. **Frequency and Volume**: Include pull-ups consistently in your workout routine. Adjust volume based on your fitness level, gradually increasing as your strength improves.

6. **Variety in Training**: Combine pull-ups with other exercises to target different muscle groups. This could include rows, lat pulldowns, and various grip variations.

7. **Progressive Overload**: Continuously challenge your muscles by increasing resistance or incorporating advanced variations like one-arm pull-ups or typewriter pull-ups.

8. **Warm-up**: Prioritize a thorough warm-up to prepare your muscles and joints for the demands of pull-ups. Dynamic stretching and shoulder mobility exercises can be beneficial.

9. **Bodyweight Control**: If bodyweight pull-ups are challenging, start with assisted variations or negative reps. As strength increases, transition to unassisted pull-ups.

10. **Rest and Recovery**: Allow adequate recovery between pull-up sessions to prevent overtraining and promote muscle repair. Listen to your body and avoid excessive strain.

Remember, individual responses to training vary, so tailor your approach based on personal fitness levels and goals. Consistency, proper form, and progressive overload are key elements in optimizing bodybuilding pull-ups for muscle development.

THE PLANK

Planks are a popular isometric exercise that targets the core muscles. To perform a plank, you maintain a push-up position with your arms straight, supporting your body weight on your forearms and toes. Key points about bodybuilding planks include:

1. **Core Engagement**: Planks primarily engage the core muscles, including the rectus abdominis, obliques, and transverse abdominis.

This helps strengthen the abdominal muscles, leading to improved stability and posture.

2. **Full-Body Workout**: While the focus is on the core, planks also engage other muscle groups, including the shoulders, back, and legs. This makes them an effective full-body exercise.

3. **Isometric Nature**: Planks are isometric exercises, meaning they involve static muscle contractions without joint movement. This helps build endurance and stability rather than promoting muscle growth.

4. **Variations**: There are several plank variations to target different muscle groups. Side planks work the obliques, while elevated or weighted planks can increase the intensity.

5. **Proper Form**: Maintaining proper form is crucial for effectiveness and injury prevention. Keep a straight line from head to heels, engage the core, and avoid letting your hips sag or rise.

6. **Duration and Sets**: The duration of a plank can vary based on fitness levels. Beginners may start with shorter durations (e.g., 30 seconds), gradually increasing over time. Sets can be repeated based on individual fitness goals.

7. **Benefits**: Regular incorporation of planks into a workout routine can lead to improved core strength, enhanced posture, and reduced risk of back pain. They also contribute to overall stability and balance.

8. **Inclusion in Bodybuilding Routines**: While planks alone may not contribute significantly to muscle hypertrophy, they are often included in bodybuilding routines as part of a comprehensive core training strategy.

Remember to consult with a fitness professional or healthcare provider before starting a new exercise routine, especially if you have pre-existing health conditions or concerns.

5 Ways To Make Your Planks Harder And More Effective

Planks are more useful than a fixed grasp. Discover many iterations of this body-twisting workout to work your entire core.

I think we've all done a plank or two at some point. A static plank might become monotonous after a while, regardless of your goals—you could be trying to keep the posture for one minute or pushing yourself to the maximum elevation.

Not that I'm against planks; I just think they're better. Your posture can be improved and your general core strength can be greatly increased with these workouts. Plus, depending on the kind of plank you perform, they can train your entire body. Doesn't it sound like a lot more fun than a static hold?

I enjoy varying up my training routine. Frequently, I start with the most fundamental exercise—in this case, a plank—and then incorporate another element. By doing this, I give my body a fun new challenge, keep it guessing, and broaden my range of exercises.

A word of caution before attempting these variations: make sure you have perfect form on both elbow and fully extended planks first. Before stepping it up a notch, you want to feel comfortable making those actions.

1. PLANK UP/DOWNS

I really enjoy doing this as a quick cardio workout in between strength training rounds. It works particularly well as an added challenge on an upper-body day. This exercise targets your triceps, back, shoulders, and chest in addition to raising your heart rate (of course along with your core).

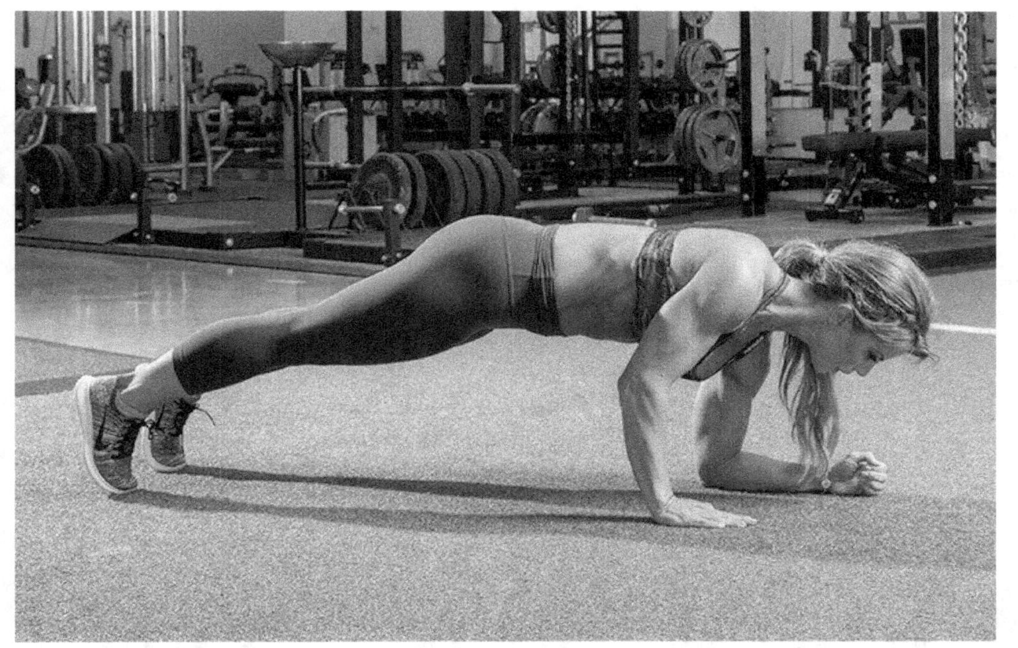

PLANK UP/DOWNS

HOW TO DO IT

- Start in the fully extended plank posture, then descend into the elbow-plank position one arm at a time.
- After a one-second pause in the elbow-plank position, push yourself back up to the fully extended plank posture, one arm at a time.
- For thirty to sixty seconds, repeat this up/down sequence. The goal of this exercise should be to quickly go from an elevated to an elbow plank, back up in a count of "1, 2, 3, 4", and then back down.

Tip: When you are lifting and lowering anything, your hips shouldn't turn. Even though you are transitioning from hands to elbows, it is important to keep your glutes tight and your spine in a neutral position throughout the exercise. You should only be moving quickly with your upper body.

2. PLANK JACKS

The plank jack, a hilarious combination of planks and the jumping jacks I hated doing in junior high physical education class, is back. It ought to be enjoyable, right? Your lower body is being worked while receiving a cardio burst exercise (imagine your glutes activating with every movement). Every repetition also works your triceps, back, shoulders, chest, and several stabilizing muscles.

There are a number different methods to execute them, and to be honest, it mostly depends on your preference, any prior injuries, and how high-impact you want your plank's "jack" motion to be. These provide an additional challenge and bonus upper body burnout exercise when added at the end of an upper-body workout (particularly in between sets of chest or shoulder movements).

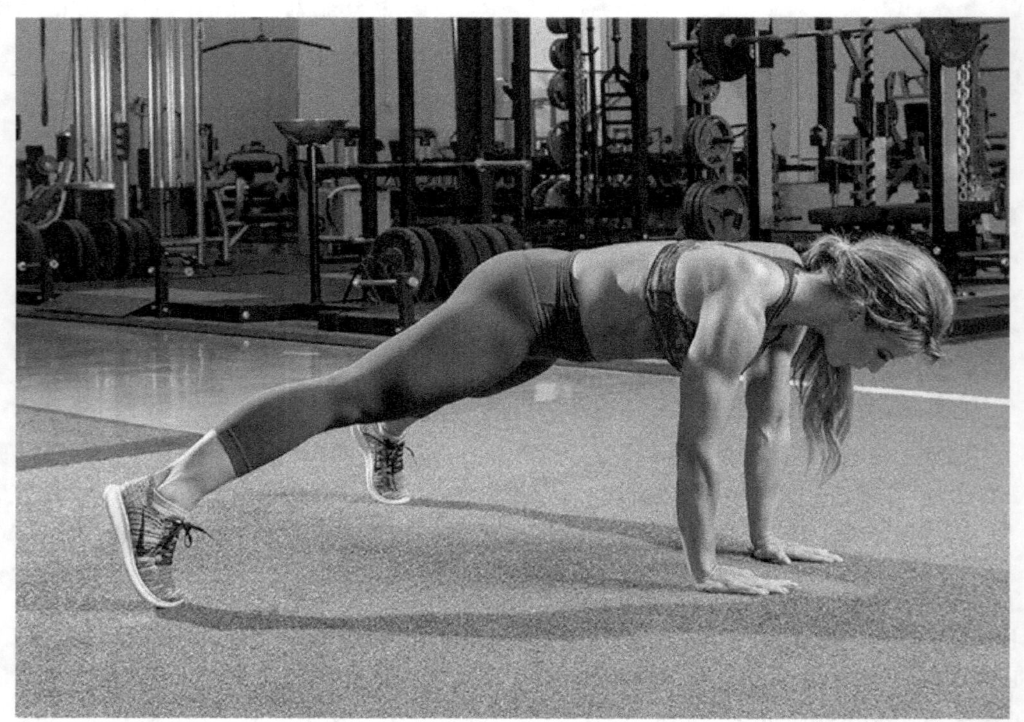

PLANK JACKS

HOW TO DO IT

- If you've never done these before, start with an elbow plank. Try them in the full-plank position if you're an intermediate or advanced practitioner. The effect on your upper body will be little less than if you go for the fully extended plank.
- Walk your right leg out to the side, walk your left leg out to the side, and then bring both back in. This is a better technique than jumping with both legs out at once.
- For the 30 to 60 seconds in each set, repeat this.

Tip: Keep your upper body still at all times. As with your legs, don't leap out with your arms. Are you looking to increase the difficulty of plank jacks? A loop band should be added somewhere above or below your knees. Your glutes and stabilizer muscles will be put to the test even more by this!

3. PUSH-UP WITH SIDE-PLANK ROTATION

These are among my all-time favorite exercises using just bodyweight! This combination is so good that I use it for in-person exercises as well as for on-the-go workouts on days when I'm at the gym. Push-ups are great for building overall strength, as we all know, so engage your complete body by combining them with a side-plank rotation. When I exercise my chest, I like to start with this combination first, even before I've completely exhausted my upper body from heavy lifting.

This push-up to side-plank rotation combination is a true full-body workout. With every push-up, your entire upper body works, your lower body works even harder while you're in the side-plank position, and your core stays active. You will also notice that your heart rate will be higher during these exercises than it would be if you were just performing a static plank.

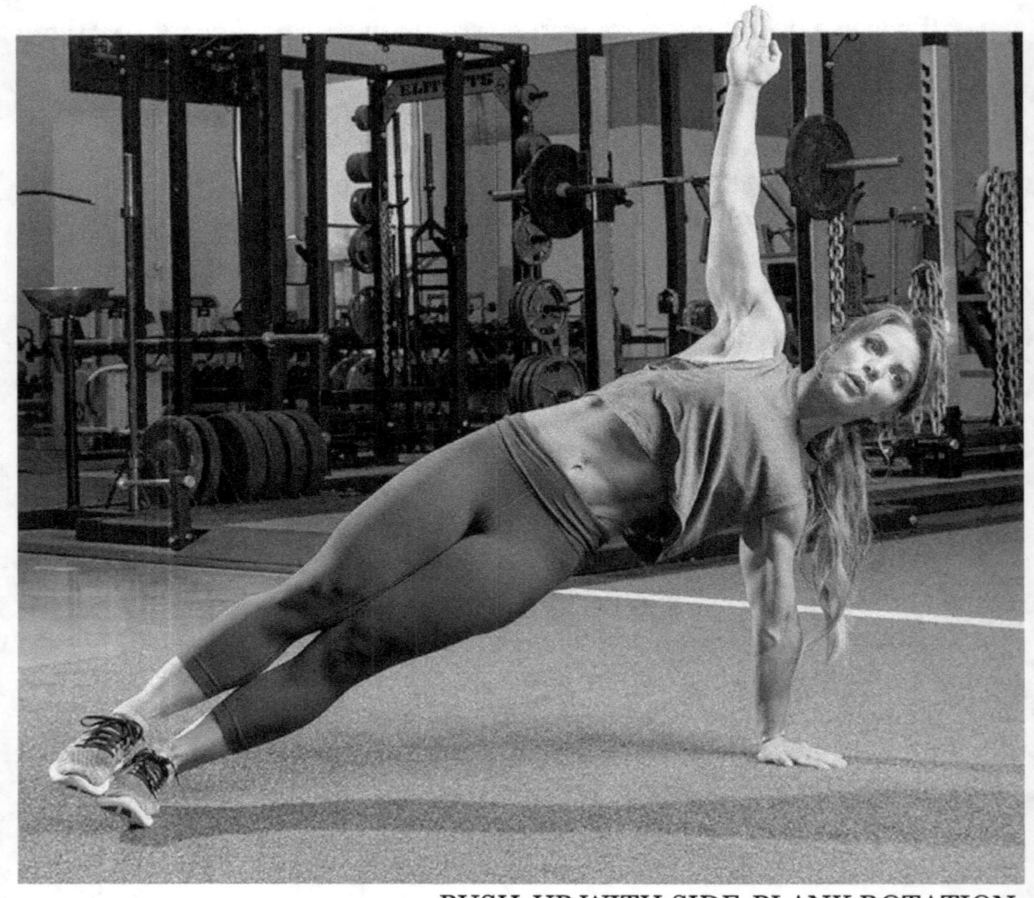

PUSH-UP WITH SIDE-PLANK ROTATION

HOW TO DO IT

- After completing one push-up, switch to a side plank.
- Perform one additional push-up and switch to the opposite side for a side plank.
- Each set, switch sides for a full minute.
- Add a push-up to side plank with leg raise once performing three to five sets at a minute starts to feel effortless.

Tip: If you think this combination is too insane, start on your knees in a modified push-up stance. From the kneeling posture, you can still execute a modified side-plank rotation. Work up to one, two, and three sets of the complete push-ups to side-plank rotations after developing your strength and coordination in this area.

4. ALTERNATING ARM-AND-LEG RAISE FROM PLANK

Here's another method to use the plank as a full-body exercise. These are my favorites to include in my core training for a fantastic lower-back and abs workout. You'll strengthen, balance, and coordination as you alternate between simultaneously extending one arm and one leg. Just keep in mind to employ opposing sides; else, balancing can become even more difficult.

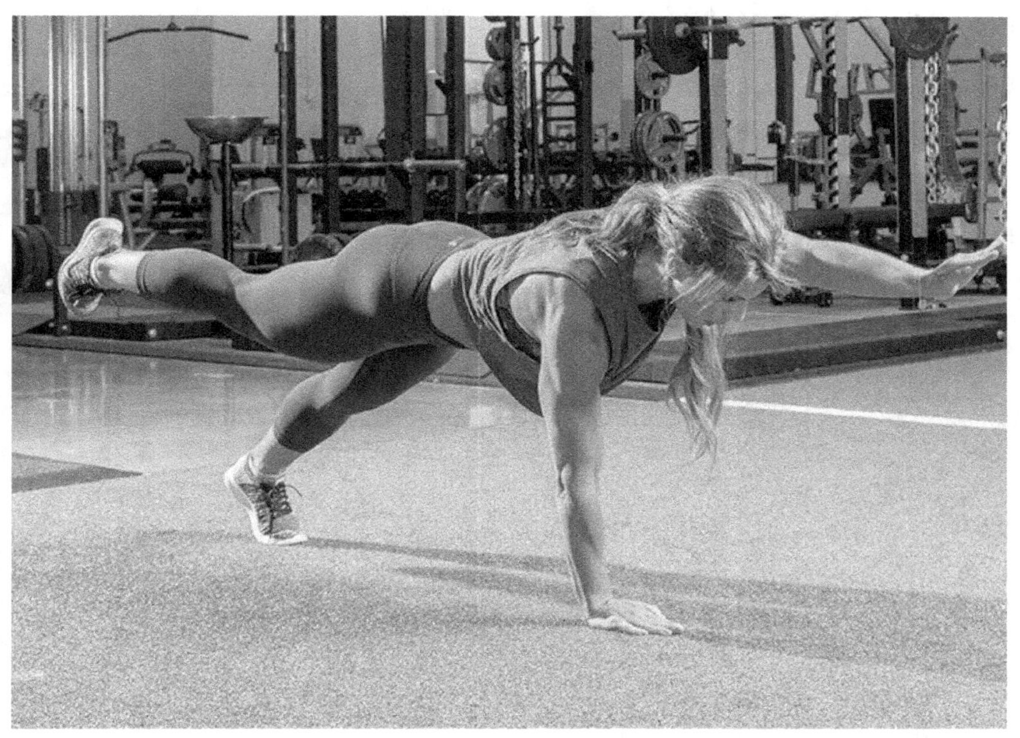

ALTERNATING ARM-AND-LEG RAISE FROM PLANK

HOW TO DO IT

- Starting from an elevated plank stance, straighten your left arm at shoulder height.
- Straighten your right leg and bring it back behind you to hip height. Maintain a taut glute and abs.
- On the other side, repeat.

Tip: If you have never done this before, start in the raised-plank position. First, extend your left arm, then bring it down. Next, extend your right leg from behind and bring it down. I frequently combine this workout with a set of decline bench reverse crunches. I add it to an at-home yoga day or use it at the end of a workout when I'm focusing on my abs.

5. SIDE PLANK ROTATION

Another enjoyable challenge are side planks. You can do this with your arms fully extended or on your elbows. Just as with the previous plank variants, you'll be working your core, but when you push through your elbow, forearm, or hand from the raised position, you'll be focusing more on your obliques. This exercise targets your glutes and inner thigh muscles in addition to testing your core, back, and obliques. Win-win!

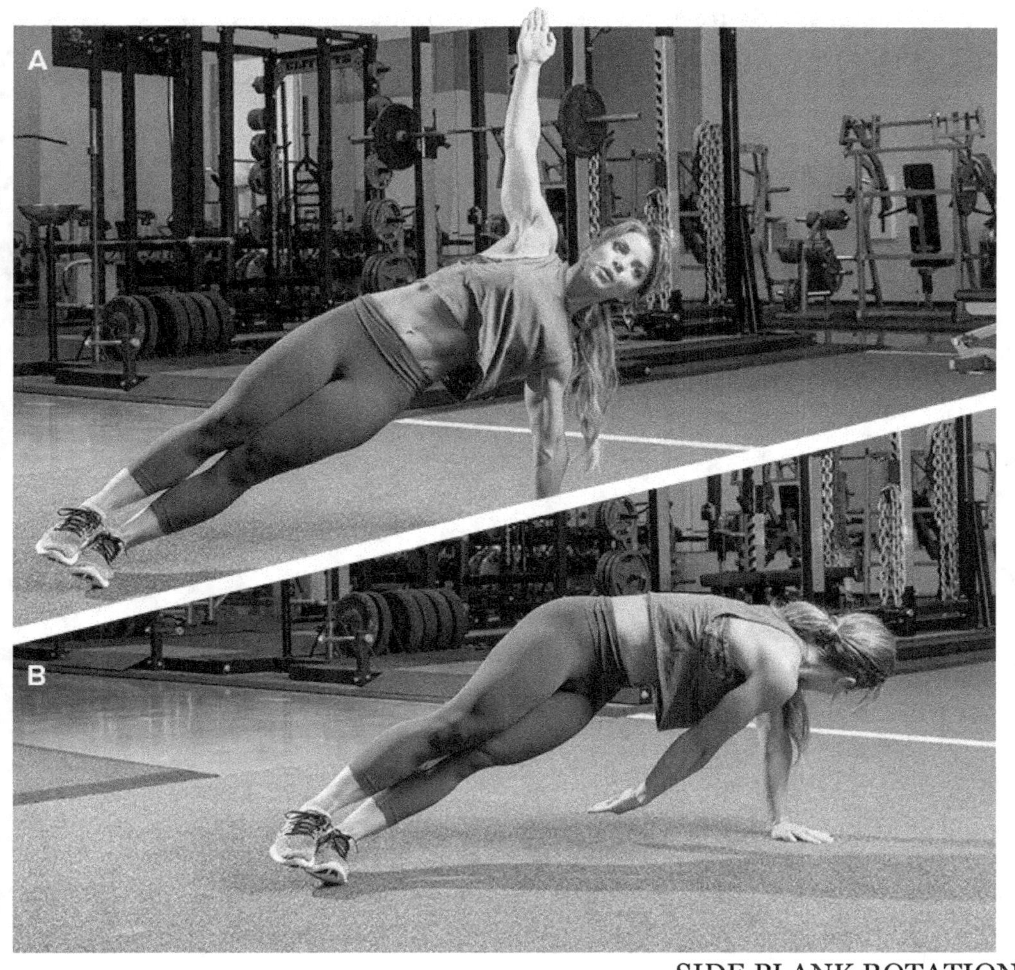

SIDE PLANK ROTATION

HOW TO DO IT

- Assume a plank posture.
- To get into a side plank position, open your shoulders and hips to the side. Hold your hips high.
- Return to starting position by rotating, but keep your upper arm extended, extending across your body to the other side.

I'll work on each side for thirty seconds, without taking a break in between. I can finish three to four complete sets in less than five minutes.

Chapter 20

YOUR BECOME THINNER LEANER STRONGER WORKOUT PLANS

All you need to start is a precise training plan to adhere to now that you know exactly how to eat and train for optimal results. Alright, let's get started.

REMEMBER THE FORMULA

Above all, you need to make sure you're using the knowledge you gained from the Become Thinner Leaner Stronger training program. Exercise regimen is not as crucial as training style. You would not achieve the maximum amount of gain if you performed the exercises in this chapter without adhering to the formula. On the other hand, you would also not achieve the best results if you used the formula but performed the incorrect workouts.

You can fully change your physique by applying the recipe consistently together with the right exercises. And you'll get that from this training program.

WARMING UP

When doing weight training, you should warm up the muscle group you'll be working before beginning your first "heavy" set.

The goal of the warm-up is to pump enough blood into the connective tissues and muscles so that they are as fully recruited as possible to do the heavier sets.

Your muscles shouldn't be fatigued throughout the warm-up. All it should do is pump circulation into them, readying the tendons and ligaments to withstand the strain of the heavier sets.

Doing this is quite simple.

Warm-Up Set 1

You should use roughly 50% of your "heavy" weight (weight that only permits 8–10 reps) for your fist warm-up set, 12 reps total, followed by a minute of rest. While you shouldn't rush this set, you also shouldn't go too slowly. It will feel really effortless and light.

Thus, if you performed three sets of nine squats with 100 pounds last week, you would begin your warm-up with 50 pounds and complete 12 repetitions before taking a minute to rest.

Warm-Up Set 2

Using the same weight as the first warm-up set, perform 10 repetitions at a slightly quicker tempo for the second set. Next, take a minute to rest.

Warm-Up Set 3

Your third set consists of six repetitions at a leisurely speed using roughly 70% of your heavy weight. It need to remain effortless and light. Your muscles should become accustomed to the hefty weights that will be used in the next two sets and this one. Once more, you should take a one-minute break after this.

Fourth to Sixth Sets:

These are your "working," or muscle-building, sets for the workout.

Proceeding to the Next Workout:

Assume for the moment that you will perform lunges. Do you need to perform an additional warm-up routine? **NO** is the response. Why would you bother when your muscles are fully warmed up and capable of handling a lot of weight?

The sole exception to this rule is if you switch from a lat pull-down to a deadlift, for example, which uses muscles that wouldn't have warmed up beforehand. You should be fine moving straight into exercises like Barbell or Dumbbell Rows, Low Rows, V-Bar Pull-downs, Weighted Pull-Ups, and so on if you warm up on the Lat Pull-down machine before beginning your back routine. However, since Deadlifts place a lot of strain on your lower back and hamstrings, you should perform a few warm-up sets to avoid straining these muscles.

YOURFIRST BECOME THINNER LEANER STRONGER TRAINING EXERCISES ROUTINES

This program asks for five days of weightlifting, two days of rest from the weights, and one day of total rest (no exercise whatsoever), along with as much cardio as you'd like to do based on your goals and what you already know.

I also have a regimen for you if you can only work out three or four days a week; I'll talk about it at the end of this chapter. Nevertheless, if you can find the time to work out five days a week, do so. That's how you'll gain the most.

What you are supposed to do is as follows:

Mon–Fri: Weight Lifting
Sat: Complete rest (No Workouts)
Sun–Tues/Weds: Cardio

This is simple and effective for most people, however alternative options include the following:

Day 1: Weight Lift & cardio
Day 2: Weight Lift
Day 3: Cardio
Day 4: Weight Lift & cardio
Day 5: Weight Lift & cardio
Day 6:Rest
Day 7: Weight Lift

Throughout the first two months, you should perform the following exercises once a week. After the first two months, I strongly advise you to get the hardcover version of this book since it will make it easier for you to look through it and complete the tasks.

The exercises should be completed in the specified order. Perform your three heavy sets after completing your warm-up sets for the first exercise (with, of course, the appropriate break in between). Proceed to the following exercise on the list, and so on.

You may feel a little uneasy during the first week as you become used to the movements and weight ranges if you have never lifted high weights or done the workouts prescribed. For the first week, feel free to work in the 10–12 or even 12–15 rep range to gain a good feel for everything. Use your warm-up sets to familiarize yourself with the movements. Next, progress into the 8–10 range in week two.

Just to remind you, bodybuilding.com has a fantastic library of videos that you can view at www.bodybuilding.com/exercise, in case you're unfamiliar with any or all of the exercises I provide in this chapter. Some videos are also available on YouTube.

I think this is a much better way to learn the exercises than looking at a few photos for each like what most books give you. So head on over to check the exercises out before you do them.

If weight loss is your goal, you should expect to lose at least 10 to 15 pounds in the first two months if you follow the exercises below, apply the formula, train hard, and eat healthily. If muscle growth is your goal, you should also expect to gain a few pounds, which will significantly improve the way your body looks.

1st Day: Chest and Abs

Warm-up and three working sets (8–10 repetitions each) comprise the flat bench press exercise.

Bench Press with an Incline Three sets of work (8–10 repetitions each)

Three working sets of incline dumbbell bench press (8–10 repetitions each)

Dips: three working sets until failure (use the helper machine if needed)

Three sets of cable crunches with a weight that allows for 15–20 repetitions each set

Leg of the Captain's Chair Raise three sets as high as you can (no weight). Air bikes (as many as you can, no weight restriction)–3 sets

One of the best workouts for growing chest is the bench press, which works every area of your chest with both flat and incline presses. Another one of my favorites is the dip, which hits your chest at an angle that weights just can't match while still providing a tremendous stretch.

The three movements listed above form the foundation of the most efficient ab regimen I've been able to devise over the years. Simple as it may be, it will shake you to your very core. What I do is proceed straight to Cable

Crunches following a set of chest exercises. After completing that, I immediately do leg raises till I fail, then I attempt air bicycles, sometimes known as "air bikes," until I fail. After two to three minutes of repose, I return to my chest. After three of these "super sets," your abs will be wailing for attention and assistance. Achieving five or six complete circuits is a sign of a superstar.

2nd Day: Back

Barbell Deadlift: Three working sets followed by a warm-up

Barbell Row: Three sets of reps

One-Arm Dumbbell Row: Three repetitions

Pulldown Lat Close-Grip: Three functional sets

This combo will train your entire back and is a terrific way to build muscle in your back.

Avoid the deadlifts if you have lower back pain. Replace the deadlifts with another "approved" exercise from the list of fantastic ones I provide at the end of this chapter for each body area.

3rd DAY: Shoulders

Three working sets followed by three seated barbell military press warm-up sets

Barbell Upright Row: Three repetitions

Side Lateral Raise: Three sets of work

Three functional sets of bent-over rear delt raise

Three "heads" make up the shoulder muscle (deltoid): the anterior (front), lateral (side), and posterior (back). You need to work every head if you want full, round shoulders, and these three exercises make sure you engage every muscle in your body.

4th Day: Legs

Barbell Squat: 3 working sets following the warm-up.

Leg Press: Three Practice Sets

Barbell Lunge: 3 sets of reps

Three functional sets of Romanian Deadlift

For developing toned, attractive legs and round, bouncy bottoms, nothing works better than Romanian Deadlifts, Lunges, and Squats. These workouts will yield a great deal of benefits for you.

Avoid the Romanian Deadlifts (RDLs) and replace them with another "approved" exercise if you suffer from lower back pain.

5th Day: Arms

Three workout sets followed by alternating dumbbell curl-warm-up sets

Triceps Pushdown: Three working sets followed by a warm-up

Barbell Curl: Three practical sets

Three sets of seated tricep press exercises

These four arm workouts are among your greatest options. If you hit these hard, your arms will look amazing!

IF YOU CAN ONLY TRAIN THREE DAYS PER WEEK, DO THIS.

Don't give up if you are unable to lift five days a week. Even though three training days a week won't be as productive as five, you can still achieve significant improvements.

For me, the most effective three-day program is this one:

First Day: Tris (6 working sets; no warm-up required) and Chest (12 working sets)

Day 2: Back (6 working sets; no warm-up required) and bis (12 working sets).

Day 3: Warm-up and 12 working sets for the legs and 12 working sets for the shoulders

Exercises that you performed earlier in this chapter are repeated. All you need to do is double them every day.

THOSE INITIAL SEVERAL WEEKS

In the initial two to three weeks, a lot of the workouts may seem a little strange to you. You may likely feel a variety of aches and stiffness as you learn your weight ranges. This is all common and only a feature of the game. However, the aches will soon go away after you find your comfort level with each activity and weight for it.

However, sharp pains during lifting indicate a problem. Never try to exert yourself through a severe discomfort. Rather, let go of the weight and examine your form. If your form is good, move on to something else.

For a few weeks, avoid the workout that was hurting you and use a pain-free exercise to strengthen the affected area. Next, give the original another go and see if it still irritates you. Don't do it then if it still does.

See a doctor if you're experiencing any severe pains as it may be a sign of anything worse.

OVER A 3-DAY WEEK

<u>Chest</u>

Press with dumbbells (flat, incline)

Barbell Bench Press (inclined, flat)

Push-Up

Dip

I switch between workouts that focus on dumbbells and those that focus on barbells. For instance, I might perform dips, flat dumbbell presses, and inclined dumbbell presses for two to three months, and then for the following two to three months, I'd perform flat bench presses, inclined bench presses, and flat dumbbell presses.

The hardest kind of chest exercise is the incline press, so I usually advise doing at least one of them in your routine.

Lastly, I've completed every chest workout imaginable and have purposefully omitted several popular exercises.

For instance, the decline variety of presses shortens the length of the rep, which means less work is done by the muscle group and is therefore less effective than the flat and incline variations. The justification for performing decline presses is that they strengthen the lower chest, although the Dip is a much better exercise for this goal because it works more muscles overall, improves balance and coordination, and stimulates the nervous system more.

Additionally, I have excluded isolation workouts like machine presses and flyes because they are not as good at building muscle as the compound motions I have suggested.

<u>Back</u>

Barbell Deadlift

Pull-Up

Chin up

Row of One-Arm Dumbbells

Row T-Bar

Bent-over row of barbells

Pull-down of the front lats

Grip Pull-down Close-Up

Cable Row Seating (wide-and-close-grip)

I urge you to incorporate the Deadlift into your routine at all times. It's the best for developing your back strength and development overall. Many people complain about lower back or knee pain, but if you take care to constantly maintain perfect form and don't hurry to handle more weight than you can lift safely, you shouldn't experience any of these problems.

Thus, you will begin most of your back exercises with deadlifts. I suggest selecting a wide-gripped exercise to work your lats and a close-grip exercise to work the middle of your back for your other two workouts. Exercises that target the entire back, including the lats, middle back, and lower back, include the pull-up, T-Bar Row, and bent-over barbell row.

Barbell Deadlift, T-Bar Row, One Arm Dumbbell Row; Barbell Deadlift, Bent-Over Barbell Row, Close-Grip Pull-down; and Barbell Deadlift, Front Lat Pull-down, Pull-Up are a few exercises that I truly adore.

Shoulders

Military Press in a Seat Barbell

Pressed Dumbbells While Seated

Arnold Dumbbell Press

Front Raise with a Dumbbell

Barbell Upright Row

Lateral Side Raise

Bend-Over Back Delt Lift

Rear Delt Lift While Seated

My preferred method of working out my shoulders is to do one easy exercise for each head, always beginning with an over-head press. The Seated Barbell Military Press is my all-time favorite exercise because it really works the anterior (front) head of the shoulder.

Although the dumbbell front raise is a useful exercise, it shouldn't be used in favor of the military or dumbbell press because those two exercises are better at building mass. The Front Raise, which may be added to the conclusion of your regular workouts to make 12 working sets, can be very beneficial in building many of the minor, supporting muscles needed for the harder lifts, especially if you're really weak at press exercises. For this exercise, I also find that a rep range of 8–10 reps works best.

Seated Barbell Military Press, Side Lateral Raise, Bent-Over Rear Delt Raise, Seated Barbell Military Press, Dumbbell Front Raise, Side Lateral Raise, Seated Rear Delt Raise, and Seated Dumbbell (or Arnold) Press, Side Lateral Raise, Seated Rear Delt Raise are the only shoulder routines I alternate through.

<u>Legs</u>

Hack Squat

Barbell Squat

Front Squat

Dumbbell Lunge

Barbell Lunge

Leg Press

Romanian Deadlift

Leg Extension

Leg Curl

Legs are really easy to work. To develop attractive, powerful legs, just do this (above).

<u>Arms (bicep)</u>

Dumbbell Curl

Straight Bar Curl

E-Z Bar Curl

Barbell Curl

All you need to work on your biceps are these exercises. You can perform the opposite exercise after beginning with a bar or dumbbell curl. I concur that the Barbell Curl and Straight Bar Curl are the greatest total bicep muscle builders.

Arms(triceps)

Close-Grip Bench Press

Seated Triceps Press

Triceps Pushdown

Lying Triceps Extension

Dip

My favorite triceps exercises are those listed above.

But I do go through each of the aforementioned activities in turn. My favorite combinations are Dips (Chest Variation) and Triceps Pushdown, Close-Grip Bench Press and Triceps Press, and Seated Triceps Press and Close-Grip Bench Press.

Abs

Cable Crunch

Air Bicycles

Captain's Chair Leg Raise

Ab Roller

Hanging Leg Raise

Decline Crunch

Flat Bench Lying Leg Raise

Being thin is, as you probably already know, the "secret" to having a nice stomach, but getting the desired lines and definition requires some ab work. Although there are countless exercises for abs that people and magazines suggest, I've limited them to the few that are listed above based on their general efficacy.

When creating your own abdominal routines, I suggest beginning with a weighted exercise (some people add weight to the Decline Crunch by gripping a plate or dumbbell, but I find this quite difficult). You may add weight to leg raise movements by snatching a dumbbell in between your feet. Two unweighted exercises performed to failure come next.

Here, my regimen is rather consistent. I perform the Captain's Chair Leg Raise, the Cable Crunch, and either the Ab Roller or Air Bicycles until I burn out.

FINAL SENTENCE

It's fairly easy, isn't it? For the first two months of the program, stick to the first regimen I gave you in this chapter.

It's time to switch up some exercises and increase your strength on those for the next two months after your first two months are over and you've had your week off. You'll get a great sense of your body's reactions and what works best for it after about a year of doing this.

Chapter 21

THE NO-BS GUIDE TO SUPPLEMENTS

"The No-BS Guide to Supplements in Bodybuilding" emphasizes practical and evidence-based advice for individuals seeking optimal results in their fitness and physique journey. It typically covers key aspects such as:

1. Protein Supplements:

Protein supplements play a crucial role in bodybuilding by providing a convenient and concentrated source of protein, essential for muscle growth and repair. These supplements often contain proteins like whey, casein, or plant-based sources, delivering amino acids that aid in the synthesis of new muscle tissue.

Whey protein, derived from milk, is quickly absorbed, making it ideal for post-workout recovery. Casein, another milk protein, is slower to digest, providing a sustained release of amino acids, beneficial for prolonged muscle support.

In bodybuilding, protein supplements help meet increased protein requirements, especially during periods of intense training. They contribute to a positive nitrogen balance, fostering an anabolic environment for muscle development. However, it's essential to combine supplements with a balanced diet to ensure overall nutritional needs are met for optimal results.

2. Creatine:

Creatine is a naturally occurring compound found in small amounts in certain foods and synthesized by the body. It plays a crucial role in providing energy for short bursts of intense physical activity, such as weightlifting or sprinting. Creatine is stored in muscles and helps regenerate ATP (adenosine triphosphate), the primary energy currency of cells.

Many athletes and fitness enthusiasts use creatine supplements to enhance performance and support muscle growth. It can also aid in recovery by reducing muscle fatigue. It's essential to stay hydrated when taking creatine, as it can increase water content in muscles.

While generally considered safe, individuals with kidney issues should consult a healthcare professional before using creatine supplements.

3. BCAAs (Branched-Chain Amino Acids):

Branch Chain Amino Acids (BCAAs) are essential amino acids, including leucine, isoleucine, and valine, crucial for protein synthesis and muscle growth. In bodybuilding, BCAAs are popular as supplements to support muscle recovery, reduce muscle soreness, and enhance endurance during workouts. Leucine, in particular, plays a key role in triggering muscle protein synthesis. Including BCAAs in your regimen may aid in preserving lean muscle mass, especially during periods of calorie restriction or intense training.

4. Pre-Workout Supplements:

A pre-workout supplement is a product designed to enhance physical performance during exercise. It typically contains ingredients like caffeine, amino acids, creatine, and vitamins. These ingredients aim to increase energy levels, improve focus, and reduce fatigue, allowing individuals to push themselves harder during workouts. It's essential to follow recommended dosages and be aware of individual sensitivities to ingredients. Consulting with a healthcare professional before incorporating supplements is advisable.

5. Multivitamins:

Multivitamins play a crucial role in bodybuilding by providing a spectrum of essential vitamins and minerals that support overall health and optimal bodily functions. These micronutrients are involved in various processes, such as energy metabolism, muscle contraction, and immune function, all of which are vital for effective workouts and recovery.

In the context of bodybuilding:

- Energy Production: B-vitamins (e.g., B6, B12) aid in converting food into energy, supporting stamina during workouts.

- Muscle Function: Minerals like calcium, magnesium, and potassium are essential for muscle contraction and proper nerve function.

- Immune System Support: Intense training can stress the immune system. Vitamins A, C, D, and zinc contribute to immune function, helping to maintain overall health.

- Recovery: Antioxidant vitamins (e.g., vitamin C, E) protect cells from oxidative stress, which can occur during intense exercise, promoting faster recovery.

While multivitamins can be beneficial, they are not a substitute for a well-balanced diet. It's important for bodybuilders to prioritize a nutrient-rich diet to meet their specific needs. Always consult with a healthcare or nutrition professional before adding supplements to your regimen, as individual requirements can vary.

6. Omega-3 Fatty Acids:

Omega-3 fatty acids, found in fish oil and certain seeds, offer several benefits for bodybuilders. They aid in reducing inflammation, supporting joint health, and promoting cardiovascular function. Additionally, omega-3s may enhance muscle protein synthesis, optimizing muscle growth and recovery. Including sources like fatty fish or supplements in your diet can contribute to overall well-being and potentially improve bodybuilding outcomes.

- Highlighting the benefits of fish oil for joint health and inflammation.

- Encouragement to consume fatty fish as a primary source.

7. Vitamin D:

Vitamin D plays a crucial role in bodybuilding as it contributes to muscle function, protein synthesis, and overall strength. It helps regulate calcium absorption, supporting bone health, which is essential for proper muscle contractions and strength during workouts. Additionally, adequate vitamin D levels may positively influence testosterone levels, potentially benefiting muscle growth. Exposure to sunlight and dietary sources like fatty fish or supplements can help maintain optimal vitamin D levels for individuals engaged in bodybuilding.

8. Individual Variability:

Individual variability in the effects of supplements in bodybuilding can be influenced by factors such as genetics, metabolism, overall health, and training routine. What works well for one person may not yield the same results for another. It's essential to consider personal differences and tailor supplement choices based on individual needs and responses. Monitoring and adjusting based on one's own body's reactions can help optimize the benefits of supplements in a bodybuilding regimen.

9. Regulatory Considerations:

Regulatory considerations for bodybuilding supplements vary by country. In the United States, the FDA regulates dietary supplements, but not as rigorously as pharmaceuticals. Manufacturers are responsible for ensuring safety and labeling accuracy. Always choose supplements from reputable companies, and consult healthcare professionals for personalized advice.

Remember, individual needs may vary, and it's crucial to consult with healthcare professionals or nutritionists before incorporating new supplements into one's routine.

Chapter 22

YOUR PHYSIQUE WILL CHANGE FROM HERE ON.

Thus... This must be it, am I right? The finish is in sight.

Not in a manner.

You're currently in the process of proving to yourself that you can change your body more quickly than you ever thought possible. Yes, it has already started. You will know for sure that you can follow the instructions in this book to construct the body of your dreams over the first three to four months of training.

Realizing that you are in charge of your body and not the other way around is quite awesome. You really can transform your body to become strong, slender, and healthy.

I can assure you that, whatever how "ordinary" you may imagine yourself to be, you are capable of creating both an incredible life and an extraordinary physique.
It's normal for your newly discovered self-assurance and pride to have a knock-on effect, encouraging you to pursue new objectives and make other life improvements.

All you need to do now is follow the route I've outlined for you, and after twelve weeks, you'll be able to look in the mirror and say, "I'm glad I did," rather than, "I wish I had."

My intention with this book is to assist you in achieving your goals.
Not only should you "get in shape," but I also want you to aim for goals that you formerly believed were unachievable. I want you to feel in charge, content, and self-assured.

We can and will succeed if we cooperate as a team.

So, before you start your metamorphosis, could you promise yourself and me that you would follow every instruction in this book to achieve your objective?

Oh, and in terms of where to go from here in terms of continuing your education, I suggest you check out Martin J. Higgins' books, Retro Physique, Beginner's Bodybuilding, Bodybuilding Workouts at Home, and any other publications of his you can obtain. They will be very beneficial to you.

In it, he addresses a plethora of new misconceptions, errors, and many more that are too many to mention or explain here, but which prevent people from achieving their desired levels of fitness and health. These are the ideal reading partners for this book, and they will expand on the understanding you already possess.

In summary, if you enjoyed Become Thinner Leaner Stronger, you'll adore Martin J. Higgins' books listed above.

Chapter 23

FAQs

Question: What's the key to staying motivated?

Answer: Set realistic goals, track progress, and vary your workouts to keep things interesting. Surround yourself with a supportive fitness community for encouragement.

Question: I go places a lot. Can I still correctly follow this program?

Answer: You have to prepare beforehand. Plan your workouts and stay in hotels that are close to decent gyms (most hotel workout areas are insufficient for the kind of training you'll be doing). This usually means leaving early in the morning or right after dinner for travelers. Simply stick to your usual regimen and remember to include your supplements.

While it can be more difficult, maintaining a diet while traveling is still possible. You can locate a health food store (such as Whole Foods) in the area in advance and make a meal plan for the visit. Take stock of your needs as soon as you arrive. You can make living a healthy, full life work if it's something you value highly enough.

To keep your strength up when traveling, try doing a bodyweight exercise in your hotel room if you can't make it to the gym.

This is what you ought to do:

Push-ups till you drop (one-handed if you can)

Take a 60-second break.

Pull-ups through failure (Bring one of those doorway installation bars.)

Take a 60-second break.

Spend 30 seconds squatting (Single-leg if feasible)

Burp for thirty seconds.

mountain climbers to their demise

Take a 90-second break.

crunches that lead to failure

Take a 60-second break.

Restart with pushups.

You'll discover that doing this for 20 to 30 minutes helps maintain your size and strength even when you are unable to lift weights.

Question: I want to get in shape, but I can't find the time to work out. How am I able to get help?

Answer: To be honest, I don't know anyone who manages to find time for exercise. "Ronald, I have too much free time these days," is something I've never heard someone say. I believe all I'll need to do to get in shape and have a nice body is a couple hours a day at the gym. How should I spend my time there?

The majority of individuals always feel as though they don't have time for anything new because of their frantic, busy lives. However, that is untrue. Despite what the majority of us would like to believe, we are not too busy to exercise.

Like you and me, those who have successfully transformed their bodies have only twenty-four hours in a day to accomplish everything. In addition, they have a family, jobs, social lives, and other responsibilities to balance. The point is, though, they just scheduled their days and fit in 45 to 60 minutes of exercise.

Some people watch TV nonstop every night. Some people get up an hour earlier every day. Others use the hour after supper that their wives spend watching their children.

The point is, I have no doubt that you can work out at that period if you truly want to.

Question: How important is rest and recovery?

Answer: Vital. Muscles grow during rest, so allow at least 48 hours between working the same muscle group and prioritize sleep for optimal recovery.

Question: I'm ill. Shall I still attempt to train?

Answer: Inspite of your strong desire, please don't. I've done this error numerous times, and it just makes the illness worse. Simply relax, heal, and resume your routine.

Question: With this program, how much weight may I gain or lose, and how quickly?

Answer: The majority of people can gain or lose up to 15 pounds in the first three months using this approach, which I have been helping people with for many years. You're gaining more fat than is essential if your weekly weight gain exceeds two pounds. You can be losing too much muscle if you're dropping more than two pounds a week, which could be problematic in the long run.

Question: A trainer I showed this book to didn't think it was very good and suggested I try something different. Is he correct?

Answer: Although I'm sure the trainer is genuinely trying to help and has the best of intentions, the majority of trainers are simply ignorant of the subject. The majority don't even know if the techniques they are teaching are the most effective or not; they are just imparting what they learnt from their textbooks, many of whom aren't even in fantastic shape themselves.

If you do as I have instructed in this book, you will experience incredible success. I promise you that. These kinds of routines are followed by tens of thousands, if not hundreds of thousands, of individuals worldwide, and their outcomes speak for themselves.

Question: Is cardio necessary for bodybuilding?

Answer: While not mandatory, incorporating cardiovascular exercise helps improve overall health and can aid in managing body fat levels.

Question: I struggle a great deal to put on muscle. Will I be able to use this program?

Answer: Yes. The idea of the "hard gainer" is something I reject. In all the years I've been playing this game, I have never seen a "hard gainer" who was genuinely eating and training correctly. Most of the time, they weren't eating enough and weren't lifting heavy enough to build maximal muscle.

I can assure you that you will put on muscle if you follow my training and nutrition recommendations. Story ends here.

Question: Can I build muscle without supplements?

Answer: Yes, but supplements can be helpful. Focus on whole foods first, and consider supplements like protein powder, creatine, and vitamins if needed.

Question: I've had trouble maintaining my exercise regimens. Why even try yours, should I?

Answer: There's nothing more frustrating than working so hard at the gym every day and not seeing any progress. This is without a doubt the main cause of people giving up on their exercise regimens. Yes, this program functions. Even better, it functions fast.

Imagine if you could shed around 20 pounds of fat and develop noticeable lean, toned muscle in just three months. What if your loved ones were always praising your appearance? People's heads begin to turn. Your acquaintances are wondering what on earth you're doing. You feel more robust and vivacious than you have in a long time.

Yes, that is definitely attainable. All you need to do is take the first step.

Question: I struggle to make wholesome meals every day of the week. How should I proceed?

Answer: One easy fix is to cook healthful meals in large quantities, portion them out, and bring them to work. You may simply put it in the microwave or toaster oven for a short while to get it ready.

When I do this, I cook a batch on Sundays and Wednesdays, preparing enough food for a few days at a time.

Question: My pals who are not in good shape always want me to eat bad foods with them. How should I proceed?

Answer: Remain alert and avoid the same mistakes that led to their initial lack of fitness.

You should be careful not to use the poor eating habits of those you are dining with as an excuse to adopt your own.

You might also attempt to motivate them to accompany you on your journey towards a more attractive, healthy, and energetic physique. Perhaps limit the times you eat with them to when you can treat yourself to a cheat meal.

Question: How often should I train each muscle group?

Answer: Aim for 2-3 times per week, allowing adequate rest between sessions to promote muscle recovery and growth.

Question: Should I focus more on high reps or heavy weights?

Answer: Both have benefits. Include a mix in your routine - heavy weights for strength and lower reps, and higher reps for muscular endurance and definition.

Question: How crucial is nutrition in bodybuilding?

Answer: Nutrition is paramount. Ensure a balanced diet with sufficient protein, carbohydrates, and healthy fats to fuel workouts and support muscle development.